Is Weight Loss Surge Right for You?

IS WEIGHT LOSS SURGERY RIGHT FOR YOU?

Robin F. Apple
James Lock
and Rebecka Peebles

OXFORD
UNIVERSITY PRESS
2006

OXFORD
UNIVERSITY PRESS

Oxford University Press, Inc., publishes works that further
Oxford University's objective of excellence
in research, scholarship, and education.

Oxford   New York
Auckland   Cape Town   Dar es Salaam   Hong Kong   Karachi
Kuala Lumpur   Madrid   Melbourne   Mexico City   Nairobi
New Delhi   Shanghai   Taipei   Toronto

With offices in
Argentina   Austria   Brazil   Chile   Czech Republic   France   Greece
Guatemala   Hungary   Italy   Japan   Poland   Portugal   Singapore
South Korea   Switzerland   Thailand   Turkey   Ukraine   Vietnam

Published by Oxford University Press, Inc.
198 Madison Avenue, New York, New York 10016

www.oup.com

Oxford is a registered trademark of Oxford University Press

Library of Congress Cataloging-in-Publication Data
Apple, Robin F. (Robin Faye)
Is weight loss surgery right for you? / Robin F. Apple, James Lock, and Rebecka Peebles
p. cm.
ISBN-13 978-0-19-531315-4
ISBN 0-19-531315-1
1. Obesity—Surgery—Popular works.   2. Gastric bypass—Popular works.   3. Weight loss—
Popular works.   I. Title.
RD540.A65 2006
617.4'3—dc22   2006007414

9 8 7 6 5 4 3 2 1
Printed in the United States of America
on acid-free paper

Contents

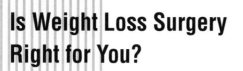

Is Weight Loss Surgery
Right for You?

Chapter 1 *Introduction*

If you are currently considering any form of weight loss surgery, it is likely that you have been thinking about your decision for some time. Certainly, it is a decision that warrants much thoughtful consideration. Hopefully this book will help you with various aspects of your decision-making process.

Perhaps you began to think about weight loss surgery after a conversation with your primary care physician, who was concerned about specific obesity-related health problems, such as heart disease, hypertension, high cholesterol, diabetes, or sleep apnea. Perhaps as weight loss surgeries of various types got more media coverage, you learned more about one or more of the procedures and thought that some form of weight loss surgery might be right for you. Possibly, a friend or relative has already undergone weight loss surgery. Or maybe you just began to research it on your own after years of struggling with more traditional methods of weight loss, typically involving dieting and exercise. In any case, you've obviously begun to think seriously about having surgery to correct your weight problem once and for all or you wouldn't be reading this.

The decision to pursue weight loss surgery should not be taken lightly. There are many factors to consider. This book contains all the need-to-know information about weight loss surgery and how to decide whether or not it is right for you. It will help guide you through the decision-making process by providing information on the various types of bariatric surgery available, their respective risks and benefits, the professional consultations and evaluations you will need to undergo prior to surgery, and what to expect postoperatively.

If you are considering weight loss surgery, this book will ensure you have all the tools necessary to make the best decisions, particularly if it is used in conjunction with ongoing counseling or psychotherapy sessions focused on relevant issues.

Chapter 2   *Is Weight Loss Surgery Right for You?*

The following issues should be taken into account as you consider whether or not weight loss surgery is right for you.

Body Weight

Determining Your BMI

You are most likely considering weight loss surgery because you are obese. But there may be medical concerns and similar factors that will sway your decision one way or the other. You will want to consider all these factors as you think about weight loss surgery.

First, do you qualify for the diagnosis of severe obesity? This is one of the first considerations when deciding if surgery is an appropriate weight loss tool for you. Doctors use the body mass index (BMI) to categorize degrees of overweight in patients. Consult Figure 2.1 to determine your BMI, or you can calculate your BMI as follows:

$$\text{BMI} = \frac{\text{weight in kilos}}{(\text{height in meters})^2} \quad \text{OR} \quad \frac{\text{weight in pounds} \times 703}{(\text{height in inches})^2}$$

Figure 2.1 Body Mass Index Chart

	Normal						Overweight					Obese					
BMI	19	20	21	22	23	24	25	26	27	28	29	30	31	32	33	34	35
Height (inches)							**Body weight (pounds)**										
58	91	96	100	105	110	115	119	124	129	134	138	143	148	153	158	162	167
59	94	99	104	109	114	119	124	128	133	138	143	148	153	158	163	168	173
60	97	102	107	112	118	123	128	133	138	143	148	153	158	163	168	174	179
61	100	106	111	116	122	127	132	137	143	148	153	158	164	169	174	180	185
62	104	109	115	120	126	131	136	142	147	153	158	164	169	175	180	186	191
63	107	113	118	124	130	135	141	146	152	158	163	169	175	180	186	191	197
64	110	116	122	128	134	140	145	151	157	163	169	174	180	186	192	197	204
65	114	120	126	132	138	144	150	156	162	168	174	180	186	192	198	204	210
66	118	124	130	136	142	148	155	161	167	173	179	186	192	198	204	210	216
67	121	127	134	140	146	153	159	166	172	178	185	191	198	204	211	217	223
68	125	131	138	144	151	158	164	171	177	184	190	197	203	210	216	223	230
69	128	135	142	149	155	162	169	176	182	189	196	203	209	216	223	230	236
70	132	139	146	153	160	167	174	181	188	195	202	209	216	222	229	236	243
71	136	143	150	157	165	172	179	186	193	200	208	215	222	229	236	243	250
72	140	147	154	162	169	177	184	191	199	206	213	221	228	235	242	250	258
73	144	151	159	166	174	182	189	197	204	212	219	227	235	242	250	257	265
74	148	155	163	171	179	186	194	202	210	218	225	233	241	249	256	264	272
75	152	160	168	176	184	192	200	208	216	224	232	240	248	256	264	272	279
76	156	164	172	180	189	197	205	213	221	230	238	246	254	263	271	279	287

Source: *The Practical Guide to the Identification, Evaluation, and Treatment of Overweight and Obesity in Adults.* National Heart, Lung, and Blood Institute and North American Association for the Study of Obesity. Bethesda, Md: National Institutes of Health; 2000. NIH Publication number 00-4084, October 2000.

Obese				Extreme obesity														
36	37	38	39	40	41	42	43	44	45	46	47	48	49	50	51	52	53	54
				Body weight (pounds)														
172	177	181	186	191	196	201	205	210	215	220	224	229	234	239	244	248	253	258
178	183	188	193	198	203	208	212	217	222	227	232	237	242	247	252	257	262	267
184	189	194	199	204	209	215	220	225	230	235	240	245	250	255	261	266	271	276
190	195	201	206	211	217	222	227	232	238	243	248	254	259	264	269	275	280	285
196	202	207	213	218	224	229	235	240	246	251	256	262	267	273	278	284	289	295
203	208	214	220	225	231	237	242	248	254	259	265	270	278	282	287	293	299	304
209	215	221	227	232	238	244	250	256	262	267	273	279	285	291	296	302	308	314
216	222	228	234	240	246	252	258	264	270	276	282	288	294	300	306	312	318	324
223	229	235	241	247	253	260	266	272	278	284	291	297	303	309	315	322	328	334
230	236	242	249	255	261	268	274	280	287	293	299	306	312	319	325	331	338	344
236	243	249	256	262	269	276	282	289	295	302	308	315	322	328	335	341	348	354
243	250	257	263	270	277	284	291	297	304	311	318	324	331	338	345	351	358	365
250	257	264	271	278	285	292	299	306	313	320	327	334	341	348	355	362	369	376
257	265	272	279	286	293	301	308	315	322	329	338	343	351	358	365	372	379	386
265	272	279	287	294	302	309	316	324	331	338	346	353	361	368	375	383	390	397
272	280	288	295	302	310	318	325	333	340	348	355	363	371	378	386	393	401	408
280	287	295	303	311	319	326	334	342	350	358	365	373	381	389	396	404	412	420
287	295	303	311	319	327	335	343	351	359	367	375	383	391	399	407	415	423	431
295	304	312	320	328	336	344	353	361	369	377	385	394	402	410	418	426	435	443

A BMI of 20–25 is considered normal, 25–30 overweight, and over 30 obese. However, surgery is not recommended as a weight management tool unless your BMI is over 40, or is over 35 and you have other significant health problems. If your BMI is under 35, that is wonderful news! This means that you are at significantly less risk from being overweight and no longer need to consider surgery, as other weight loss methods may well succeed and will carry less risk.

If your BMI is over 40, you are severely, or morbidly, obese, and surgery may be an option worth considering. In the few studies that have examined weight loss surgery and compared it to traditional weight loss methods, bariatric surgery seems to result in greater weight loss over time in patients who are significantly overweight. A description of the different types of surgeries and more detail on the research is given in the following chapters.

If your BMI is between 35 and 40, or if you haven't had a good health screening in a while, the next step is to assess your overall health, paying particular attention to conditions that result primarily from or are greatly exacerbated by being overweight. It is important to ask your doctor for a comprehensive history and exam. Some overweight patients hate to go to the doctor because they feel self-conscious and sometimes even feel that the doctor's office is not a friendly place. If this is the case, be sure to ask friends to recommend a doctor you feel comfortable with and trust. You deserve to have a provider you enjoy seeing. Considering bariatric surgery is a big step and it will help if you can discuss it openly with your physician.

Being overweight can affect almost every organ in your body. Table 2.1 lists most of the conditions that can adversely affect your health and are often caused or worsened by being significantly overweight.

Table 2.1 Illnesses and Conditions Worsened by Obesity

Organ/System	Illness	Diagnostic Tests	Abnormal Levels
Cardiac	Hyperlipidemia	Blood tests	LDL >130–160, dependent on risk factors HDL <40 cholesterol >180–200 triglycerides >150–200
	Hypertension	Blood pressure reading	Systolic blood pressure >120–139 or diastolic blood pressure >80–89
	Heart disease (coronary artery disease, heart attack, stroke, congestive heart failure)	Specialized testing; ask your doctor	Family history, abnormal tests, active symptoms, personal history of heart attack, stroke, or heart failure
	Metabolic syndrome	Presence of 3 or more abnormal levels	Abdominal obesity, high triglycerides, low HDL, high blood pressure, high fasting glucose
Endocrine	Type 2 diabetes	Blood tests	Nonfasting glucose >200 with symptoms, fasting glucose >126, 2-hour glucose (after glucose load) >200

(continued)

7

Table 2.1 (*continued*)

Organ/ System	Illness	Diagnostic Tests	Abnormal Levels
Endocrine (*continued*)	Polycystic ovarian syndrome	Physical exam, personal history, and/or labs	Menstrual irregularity and some sign of androgen excess (acne, extra hair growth in unwanted areas, overweight, and/or abnormal blood values)
Pulmonary	Obstructive sleep apnea	gram (sleep study)	Abnormal sleep study
	Restrictive lung disease & obesity hypoventilation syndrome	Lung-function testing, polysomnogram	Restrictive lung function, buildup of carbon dioxide in the blood, excessive sleepiness, signs of heart failure over time
	Asthma Polysomno-	History, physical exam, lungfunction testing	Obstructive lung function
Gastrointestinal	Fatty liver disease	Lab tests, ultrasound	Elevated liver function, abnormal ultrasound or biopsy
	Reflux or heartburn	History, physical exam; tests often unnecessary	Mild burning sensation in chest or stomach, acid taste in mouth after meals
	Gallstones	Physical exam, ultrasound	Periodic abdominal pain, gallstones seen on ultrasound
Orthopedic	Knee, back, and hip disease	X-rays, physical exam, MRI when necessary	Abnormal range of motion, chronic pain, abnormal radiologic tests

Organ/ System	Illness	Diagnostic Tests	Abnormal Levels
Brain	Idiopathic intracranial hypertension	Comprehensive eye exam, visual fields testing, lumbar puncture; MRI may be indicated	Persistent headaches, blind spots in vision, elevated spinal-fluid pressure
Genito-urinary	Stress incontinence	History	Incontinence while laughing, coughing, sneezing
	Gout	History, physical exam, labs	Joint inflammation, high uric-acid level in the blood
Skin & Blood Vessels	Infections	Physical exam	Red skin with an odor, especially in skinfolds and creases: under the breasts, beneath the abdomen, in leg skin folds; fungal infections of the nails, poor wound healing due to poor circulation in the extremities
	Varicose veins	Physical exam	Dark purple veins on the lower legs
	Deep venous thrombosis	Physical exam, ultrasound	
Cancer	All organs, but especially prostate, colon, breast, uterus	Multiple modalities	Abnormal test results

Cardiac Risk

Hyperlipidemia is a common complication of obesity. Studies have shown coronary artery disease, evidenced by plaques in the blood vessels extending from the heart, occurring as early as late adolescence. They have also shown that high LDL ("bad") cholesterol, low HDL ("good") cholesterol, and high triglycerides are common factors accompanying the development of coronary artery disease. As a result, all obese adults should be screened for lipid or cholesterol abnormalities. Lifestyle changes are often the first line of therapy against abnormal lipids in the blood. Hypertension is also increasingly recognized as a common side effect of obesity. Weight loss can produce dramatic improvements in blood pressure.

If you have been diagnosed with obesity, hypertension, and hyperlipidemia, you may also have "the metabolic syndrome." This is a newly described clustering of metabolic risk factors, known to have a significant negative effect on heart health. The factors include abdominal obesity, low HDL, high triglycerides, insulin resistance or diabetes, and high blood pressure. All these factors are thought to be caused by insulin resistance, a condition in which the body becomes increasingly resistant to the actions of insulin, a hormone secreted by the pancreas.

If you have had chest pain or shortness of breath your doctor may have tested you for the possible presence of arteriosclerosis, or coronary artery disease. If you have noticed any of these symptoms and have not told your doctor, you should call him or her immediately, as they can be signs of serious illness. If you have had a heart attack, stroke, or congestive heart failure, you have certainly been told that your weight may be contributing to your poor heart health.

Type 2 Diabetes/Glucose Intolerance

The incidence of type 2 diabetes in the United States is rising dramatically, paralleling the rise in obesity. Obesity is a known contributor to the development of type 2 diabetes. Other risk factors include a positive family history of NIDDM (noninsulin-dependent diabetes), increased body fat and abdominal fat, insulin resistance, and ethnicity (with greater risk in African American, Hispanic, and Native American adults). Heart disease, vision problems, kidney failure, high blood pressure, and stroke can complicate NIDDM. Because NIDDM can lead to premature death and disability, addressing excess weight in people with type 2 diabetes is critical.

Polycystic Ovary Syndrome and Menstrual Irregularities

First of all, ovarian cysts are normal variants for many women. Having cysts on your ovaries does not mean you have polycystic ovary syndrome (PCOS). Many women suffer from PCOS, which is characterized by menstrual changes, acne, or excessive hair growth (on the face, abdomen, chest, and back)—signs of hyperandrogenism, or excessive male hormones. About 50–75% of women with PCOS are obese, and obesity may be a factor in the development of PCOS in some susceptible women. If you have been diagnosed with PCOS and are obese, you have an elevated risk of developing hyperlipidemia, hypertension, diabetes, and the metabolic syndrome. It may also be especially hard for you to lose weight because many women with this syndrome have abnormalities in insulin metabolism. To complete this negative health cycle, obesity seems to contribute to the insulin resistance and risk for diabetes that many women with PCOS experience.

Pulmonary Risk and Obstructive Sleep Apnea

Obstructive sleep apnea (OSA) is common among the extremely obese. This condition has a known link to future cardiovascular disease and can be fatal. Current recommendations state that all overweight adults should be screened for snoring, and those who snore should have a sleep study including a polysomnogram to determine if they have OSA.

Many overweight individuals are diagnosed with asthma. Obesity is certainly one of many factors that can worsen symptoms of asthma. However, sometimes shortness of breath indicates that there is either undiagnosed heart disease or that extra weight is making it harder for the lungs to do their job every day. This is not asthma but restrictive lung disease. It is helped not by inhalers but by weight loss. So if you have shortness of breath and you haven't talked to your doctor, make sure to do so to clarify the specific cause is, whether or not you already know you have asthma.

In severe cases, the restriction that excess weight puts on the lungs can lead to something called obesity hypoventilation syndrome, a condition in which blood oxygen decreases and carbon dioxide increases, all because the lungs are unable to function optimally. This condition can lead to daytime sleepiness and over the long term can cause congestive heart failure.

Gastrointestinal Problems

Many kinds of gastrointestinal problems can occur in significantly overweight people. Nonalcoholic fatty liver disease (NAFLD) is currently the most common cause of abnormal liver tests in the United States. It is commonly seen in association with obesity, diabetes, hypertension, and hypertriglyceridemia. Most patients have no symptoms and present only with mildly abnormal laboratory results. It is not clear how NAFLD develops, but it can progress to hepatitis, cirrhosis, and end-stage liver disease. In one study examining the liver biopsies of morbidly obese adults preparing to undergo gastric bypass surgery, 65% of the patients had moderate to severe liver changes, 12% had advanced fibrosis, or scarring of the liver, and 33% had nonalcoholic hepatitis. The presence of type 2 diabetes was strongly correlated with advanced liver disease, more so than was BMI.

Gastrointestinal reflux, or heartburn, is a common but bothersome condition that is often exacerbated by weight. Reflux can cause chest pain, an acid taste in the mouth, and a cough, among other symptoms. Fatty foods, cigarettes, alcohol, caffeine, and certain medications can worsen it. While reflux can often be managed medically, it can sometimes lead to changes in the esophagus that can predispose one to cancer.

Finally, nearly 50% of cases of gallstones, small stones that can obstruct the normal flow of bile from and within the gall bladder, are associated with obesity. Gallstones can impede efforts at weight loss. Also, gallstones can sometimes be a complication of weight loss surgery as well. Be on the lookout for this condition, which often causes periodic abdominal pain, particularly if you have a family history of gall bladder disease, in order to get diagnosed and treated early.

Orthopedic Complications

Overweight adults are at increased risk for a number of weight-related orthopedic complications. Chronic excess weight can lead to a bowing of the lower legs called Blount's disease. Significant hip, knee, and back pain, and even osteoarthritis can result from the excess pressure on joints that increased body mass imposes. Many overweight patients require hip and knee replacements that, while effective, are costly and time-consuming interventions to manage pain and improve range of motion. Significant weight loss is known to help with such orthopedic disease.

Idiopathic Intracranial Hypertension (Pseudotumor Cerebri)

Idiopathic intracranial hypertension (IIH), also known as pseudotumor cerebri, is a condition seen much more commonly in obese individuals. As its name implies, IIH is associated with increased intracranial pressure in the absence of tumors or other brain disease. It often causes severe headaches and can sometimes lead to blindness. To diagnose IIH, your doctor will need to do a careful eye exam and perhaps even use magnetic resonance imaging (MRI) and a spinal tap, or lumbar puncture, to check the pressure of your spinal fluid. Once diagnosed, IIH that requires that you promptly lose weight.

Genitourinary Conditions

Many overweight women experience stress incontinence, a condition that can cause mild to severe leakage of urine from the bladder when they sneeze, laugh, cough, or even go for a walk. The condition develops when the abdomen increasingly exerts pressure on the bladder. Although surgery and medications can help control the problem, they often fail to. Weight loss can often significantly relieve symptoms.

Gout is caused by a buildup of uric acid that exceeds what the kidneys can filter. The acid builds up in the joints and can cause swelling, inflammation, and pain, most commonly in the big toe or ankle joints. Obesity increases the risk of developing gout, as does alcohol consumption, a diet high in uric acid (red meat, red wine, cream sauces), and kidney failure. Recent studies describe links between gout and high blood pressure as well. While gout is best managed with dietary changes and medication, weight loss will help prevent its recurrence.

Skin and Blood Vessels

Often, overweight patients notice that areas of hanging skin folds, particularly around the breasts, abdomen, and inner thighs, can become chafed, irritated, and difficult to clean. Superficial fungal or bacterial infections of the skin can result and can lead to deep tissue infections, although this is rare. Patients who are extremely obese, especially those with diabetes, tend to have decreased circulation to their hands and feet, delaying the healing of such infections.

Obese individuals often develop venous stasis, wherein slowed blood flow to the legs' veins leads to damage to the valves in the leg veins. Obesity can worsen this condition by making it hard to maintain regular mobility: a sedentary lifestyle further inhibits blood flow. Especially in those with a family history of venous stasis, this can lead to superficial varicose veins, a benign but unattractive condition. A separate, more serious complication of venous stasis is deep venous thrombosis (DVT), a blood clot in a deep leg vein. These clots need to be promptly managed, as they can lead to life-threatening complications such as pulmonary embolism. Leg swelling and pain can indicate DVT.

Cancer

Cancer risk increases with obesity. It is unclear whether weight loss can decrease the risk. Cancers associated with weight gain are those of the prostate, colon, breast, uterus, and gall bladder.

Do You Qualify Medically as a Potential Surgery Candidate?

Figure 2.2 provides the equation for calculating your BMI and indicates how BMI relates to candidacy for bariatric surgery. If you do meet the criteria for clinically significant obesity (i.e., you have a BMI of 35–40 or more), and also suffer from one or more of the above health problems, you may be a good candidate for weight loss surgery. On the other hand, if you have physical or mental health problems serious enough to potentially interfere with a successful surgery, your operation may be postponed until these issues are resolved. For some extremely obese people, it may be necessary to lose at least some (or even a considerable amount of) weight before surgery can be considered safe.

Figure 2.2 Your BMI and Bariatric Surgery

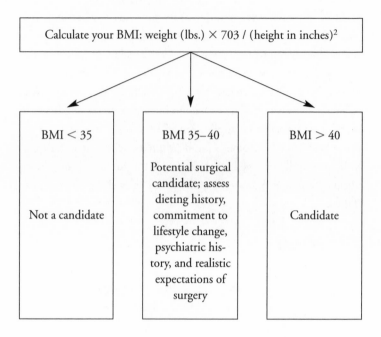

Calculate your BMI: weight (lbs.) $\times$ 703 / (height in inches)^2

BMI < 35	BMI 35–40	BMI > 40
Not a candidate	Potential surgical candidate; assess dieting history, commitment to lifestyle change, psychiatric history, and realistic expectations of surgery	Candidate

In addition to the weight criteria detailed above, the National Heart, Blood, and Lung Institute guidelines recommend that patients consider weight loss surgery only if they are at high risk for obesity-associated conditions and if they have failed at less-invasive methods of weight loss. Your doctors and surgeon should always help you determine whether the benefits of surgery outweigh the risks in your case. Most surgical programs require patients to have formally participated in a medically supervised diet and physical activity program for six months or longer before they can be determined to have "failed" at a lifestyle-change method of weight loss. Your physicians need to also assess that you understand what the surgery entails, are able to adhere to the dietary changes required postoperatively, have no significant untreated psychiatric illness that would interfere with your goals, and have demonstrated the ability to observe medical recommendations over time (www.nhlbi.nih.gov/guidelines/obesity/ob_gdlns.htm). Additional considerations include smoking history and compliance with birth control recommendations for women of childbearing age, as it is not recommended that one become pregnant for at least a year after surgery. These recommendations may seem stringent, but it is critical that patients undergoing surgery are able to fully understand what they are getting into. The lifestyle and dietary changes that surgery requires are considerable, and it can be at best defeating and at worst dangerous to fail to comply with the prescribed postoperative routine.

With the right candidate, however, surgery can be a profoundly useful tool for weight loss. There are many studies of weight loss surgery, but only a handful of studies compare surgery to conventional nonsurgical weight loss methods. These studies do seem to suggest that surgery can lead to greater overall weight loss that is sustained over significantly longer periods of time. This book is meant to help you determine if surgery would be helpful for you.

Other Issues to Consider Before Surgery

Once medical illnesses and risks have been examined thoroughly, it is important to examine your history of dieting attempts, unhealthy eating patterns and substance-abuse habits, and emotional issues before proceeding with surgery.

Dieting History

Discuss with your therapist your dieting experiences and how these experiences have affected your decision to undergo weight loss surgery.

Have your made concerted efforts over a period of several months to a year or more to try to follow one or more traditional, medically supervised weight control programs such as a modified fast (Optifast, Medifast), Weight Watcher's, a dietician-prescribed low-calorie diet, diet medications (Phen-fen, Meridia, Xenical, Redux), Jenny Craig, or Nutrisystem, or other weight loss programs such as Atkins, Slim Fast, calorie counting plus exercise, and the like? If so, how many times have you tried to diet, and for how long each time? How many pounds have you been able to lose each time, and how long were you able to keep the weight off?

If you are a teenager, your parents can offer doctors much important information about your weight and eating history. Often, weight gain starts quite young, and early eating and feeding patterns can be important in understanding how your body uses and stores energy. You should therefore expect that your parents will be asked to meet with your doctors, and you should be appreciative of their involvement in the process, even though it may, at times, seem to be the opposite of what you want.

Emotional Issues

Third, it is important to examine your emotional life, both current and past, and of course to discuss any emotional issues with your therapist as you prepare yourself to make a decision about surgery.

For obvious reasons, it is important that you are in a positive frame of mind when you undergo surgery. This means that you must not be suffering from serious depression, particularly depression that prevents you from being up, active, and optimistic about your life situation. If you are experiencing sadness or a low mood and have difficulty enjoying pleasant events and activities, or if you have had trouble getting up in the morning, are easily distracted, have poor concentration, are tearful, or have thought or planned to harm yourself or end your life, you are too depressed to proceed with surgery at this time. Similarly, anyone with significant anxiety (e.g., worries that prevent you from leaving the house, interacting comfortably with other people, or tolerating various types of fairly common daily experiences) will probably be ruled out for surgery until the anxiety can be better controlled.

Trauma

Many people who become obese have histories of traumatic experiences of one type or another, and these issues should be addressed in some form of therapy or counseling before weight loss surgery is seriously considered or the preparation process begun.

For example, trauma might have occurred as the result of abandonment or early abuse—physical, verbal, or sexual; early illness or prior surgical complication; or exposure to other extreme situations of one type or another. Trauma, especially when untreated, can result in the traumatized individual's having a shaky sense of himself or herself both physically and emotionally. One traumatic experience often leaves individuals vulnerable to subsequent trauma in other difficult circumstances, especially those that might involve physically invasive procedures, even when such bodily "assaults" take the form of an invited and highly desired surgery. An elective surgery, or any surgery for that matter, involves trauma to the body in the form of a wound, an alteration of structure and of function, and an unpredictable outcome, including various risks and potential untoward side effects or consequences. Because of this, any individual with a trauma history, particularly a recent trauma or a trauma for which he or she has never received help, should get psychological treatment specific to resolving those issues before seriously considering weight loss surgery. With the fresh perspective that often accompanies therapy, on the meaning and impact of the past trauma, the person might opt in the end to delay or to forego weight loss surgery altogether.

Alcohol and Substance Abuse or Dependence

Also, if you are currently using any type of substance (such as drugs, alcohol, or a combination of both) to cope with depression, anxiety, or other problematic moods (e.g., possibly as a form of "self-medication") it is not wise to schedule your surgery at this time. If you have been sub-stance-free for three to five years (the typical recommendation of surgical teams) yet are prone to rely on other, problematic strategies to regulate your mood, it is best to address these issues in therapy before undergoing weight loss surgery. For example, if you drink alcohol to excess (or have a strong need for two or more alcoholic beverages every day and/or experience "side effects" from drinking too much, such as drunkenness, difficulty getting up in the morning, problematic interactions with other people, blackouts, etc.), regularly smoke marijuana, use any type of "upper" (cocaine, "crank," or other amphetamines) or any licit or illicit type of "downer" (heroin, valium, etc.), you need to address these substance abuse concerns before surgery. In some cases, your medical team may recommend that you join Alcoholics Anonymous or Narcotics Anonymous. Inpatient or residential treatment may be appropriate when there is a physical dependency on alcohol or drugs.

In addition to taking stock of your problems with drugs and alcohol, your doctors will also ask you about your cigarette-smoking habits. In most instances, you will be asked to stop smoking cigarettes several months before surgery or cautioned to forego the operation, because smoking can complicate recovery and healing.

Binge Eating, "Grazing," Purging, and Other Problematic Eating Behaviors

While some obese individuals report problematic eating behaviors such as out-of-control binge eating, eating a lot very late at night, grazing throughout the day, or taking in excessive amounts of regular soda, many report simply eating too much at regular meals and snacks and exercising too little.

If you have a problem with binge eating, it definitely needs to be addressed before surgery for a number of reasons. Binge eating is defined as eating a large amount of food (e.g., more than others would consume in a similar circumstance) in a small amount of time in a manner that feels "out of control" or irresistible and impossible to interrupt. Some people who binge report a sense of "spacing out" or dissociating while they are eating. For example, while eating, they might be able to block out their thoughts and feelings in full or to some degree, making overeating a seemingly "great escape" from all types of distress. About half of those who are obese have problems with binge eating. If you frequently binge (perhaps in addition to other forms of overeating), it is best that you try to resolve that problem before undergoing surgery.

While there is no research stating definitively that binge eating undermines the outcomes of all bariatric surgery procedures, in some cases the behavior may lead to postoperative problems, including eventual weight re-gain. It is important to keep in mind that weight loss surgery will not by itself solve the problem of binge eating, even though it may be more difficult to overeat after surgery. In fact, binge eating, while not substance abuse per se, can be thought of as similarly addictive—a form of emotion regulation particularly common among individuals with significant weight problems. So, rather than continuing to rely on overeating as one of your primary tools of mood regulation, it is best to develop a repertoire of alternative tools in advance of the surgery.

If you have been purging, depending on the extent and type of purging and how recently you purged, your team may recommend that you delay your surgery. Typically, regular purging is associated with emotional distress of one type or another and is considered a poor prognostic sign for surgery; it can also be associated with various types of psychological distress.

While some of the above discussion might intimidate or discourage you, it is included to remind you of the seriousness of your decision to undergo weight loss surgery. Be assured that the professionals with whom you will be working are all on your side—they are doing their job of rigorously evaluating your fitness for surgery in order to help you make the best decision you can by fully considering all of your needs and issues.

Remember that neither your surgeons nor the mental health professionals working with you are invested in withholding any weight loss surgery procedure from you or any other appropriate candidate, although to someone whose surgery is rejected or postponed, it can feel this way. Many individuals who have struggled with mild to moderate depression or have a past history of more serious depression are approved for surgery and are even encouraged in it when the issue of obesity is seen as significantly contributing to their depression. Similarly, those who have resolved past problems with substance abuse and have been free and clear of their addictions for years may be accepted for surgery as long as there are no other concerns. In the end, what your therapist and the other members of the surgical team look for is evidence that you have worked on and resolved your problems with the assistance of some type of counseling (e.g., group treatment, psychotherapy, or other treatment), and that you are continuing to do so in your current therapy.

Social Support

Another factor that may play a role in how you are viewed as a surgical candidate is the level of social support available to you.

Those who tend to have the best surgical outcomes have a social support and resource network that is accessible at all stages of the process: for example, during preparation for surgery, while undergoing the procedure, during the initial healing and recovery phase, and in later stages of adjustment, including coming to terms with the necessary long-term lifestyle changes. Significant others living with you or providing the most support to you should be behind your decision to undergo the procedure. They need to support you in all aspects of your new eating and activity patterns. They should help you keep appropriate foods in your home and refrain from pushing you to eat more than you need, encourage exercise and any "incidental" physical activities, and congratulate you on your successes.

Having adequate social support also means that there are significant others available to visit you and take care of you in the first days after your procedure, when you will be in need of some solid "cheerleading." You will have undergone a procedure that involved a certain degree of pain, discomfort, and disorientation. Also, you will be facing the need to make significant changes in your eating patterns, your relationship to food, and your life in general, including how you relate to others—particularly if socializing often involved food. For example, if you have friends with whom you regularly "splurge" or systematically overeat, you will need to change the dynamics of those relationships so that there is no one around who can sabotage your progress by engaging you in old, familiar, but dysfunctional patterns. In the extreme case, it might be necessary to alter your network of social contacts to exclude those likely to undermine your progress and success.

Although it is true that everyone needs social support to undergo bariatric surgery, if you are a teenager, this is especially important. As you know, you depend on your parents for food, shelter, and often for transportation. As a result, it is imperative that your parents fully agree with you regarding weight loss surgery. In addition, your parents' ability to support you must be assessed. They will have to demonstrate their understanding, commitment, and ability to follow through on recommendations, just as you will.

When contemplating weight loss surgery, many individuals decide to join a weight loss surgery support group in addition to getting individual counseling. Typically, in any community where a weight loss surgery program is offered, there will be at least one support group available to people both before and after they undergo a procedure. In addition, several "chat rooms" have sprung up on Web sites that address obesity issues. While face-to-face support is important, augmenting this support through a chat room or other Internet community can be helpful for some individuals, particularly those who have limited mobility or are geographically remote.

As a teenager, you may feel that you have little to gain from attending support groups populated mostly by adults who have had or may have the surgery. Although this is an understandable sentiment, you should really reconsider. Even if you decide not to share that much about yourself, just listening to those in the group can provide you with a wealth of real-world experience with the realities of bariatric surgery and postsurgical issues. You will hear about failures and successes, and you are likely to meet at least one adult with whom you have enough in common to talk to them more personally than with the group as a whole. So, don't dismiss these support groups, even if they are adult-focused, until you've tried them a few times. You might be surprised.

Commitment to Permanent Lifestyle Change

Weight loss surgery is as "nonmagical" as any diet or exercise program you have already tried, although it should significantly help you resolve your weight problem if you comply with all the recommendations. What this means is that, while the surgery will leave you with a "smaller stomach" that will alter the way you perceive food and the way your body handles it (e.g., feeling full more quickly, eliminating food more quickly, and possibly craving certain more healthy foods), it will ultimately be up to you to make the long-term surgical outcome—radical weight loss and weight loss maintenance—a successful one. This will entail a deep commitment to permanently changing the aspects of your lifestyle that contributed to your becoming obese in the first place.

You might have thought at times that you were destined or doomed to be overweight. However, even if a biological predisposition to obesity was inherited from your parents, your eating habits and activity patterns have played a significant role. Deciding that you will make a commitment to eat healthfully and nutritiously and exercise regularly is the key to ensuring long-term success with your surgery. Without this level of commitment to your future as a thinner and healthier person, the probability of your maintaining a healthy weight is low. If you can't honestly look yourself in the mirror and affirm your commitment to making these changes and improvements for the rest of your life, your hopes and expectations regarding the surgery are likely to be unrealistic. You need to address these issues as you prepare for your surgery.

If you are a teenager, recognizing that you are making a permanent lifestyle change may be even harder because you have not had many years by which to judge such a decision. It is not unusual for teenagers to want to change things right now, and having to be patient can be difficult. When making a decision about bariatric surgery, you should not rush, no matter how enthusiastic you are about proceeding. Your parents and doctors will likely seem incredibly slow and hesitant about moving forward, but they are usually acting in your best interest. It takes time to assess your ability to make the permanent changes in your lifestyle, and you will be asked to demonstrate this ability before surgery. In addition to your doctors and parents, your therapist can help you think through the kind of future you can anticipate.

Realistic Expectations

It is important that you have realistic expectations as you anticipate losing a significant amount of weight—as opposed to idealized notions about how massive weight loss will change your life. First, losing weight, even with the "assistance" of weight loss surgery, is very, very difficult. While the surgery will help you better manage your hunger and to some extent put a cap on the amount of food you can actually eat, the difficulty of preparing for and recovering from surgery is considerable. The behavioral and emotional changes you need to make to maintain new lifestyle habits that will sustain your weight loss require a great deal of effort. While you might think that you will feel great once you begin to lose weight after surgery, the reality is that at times you may feel bad. For example, your altered relationship with food and eating might lead to feelings of sadness, loss, and a sense of "not knowing what to do" during those times when you were used to dealing with your feelings by eating.

Finally, even with radical weight loss, it is quite likely that you may look and feel somewhat different than the idealized "thin version" of you that you had in mind. For example, if you were thin at an earlier point in your life, your body might "carry" thinness at this stage of life very differently. Just the effects of aging and "gravity" will change how your body will look and feel after you lose weight post-surgery. Not only might your body appear much different than you expected, but you might also have an excess amount of loose skin. Although this can be corrected to some extent with optional plastic surgery later on, it might in the meantime get in the way of your feeling as thin and fit as you expected to feel after your weight loss. Finally, even very significant weight loss will not ensure certain changes in your personality or personal life that you have been hoping for. For these, you have to work on aspects of yourself that go beyond your physical appearance and your weight.

Again, if you are a teenager, some of your hopes and expectations about bariatric surgery might be overly optimistic. As a teen, you are faced with many images—in magazines, movies, and advertisements—of the way you are supposed to look and act. As a teenager struggling with obesity, the negative impact of these idealized images is likely even greater. It is understandable to hope for drastic weight and body shape change, but the reality is that bariatric surgery does not accomplish this kind of change. Instead, surgery can help you become more physically healthy and start you on your way to making the kinds of lifestyle changes that will allow you to sustain a healthy body weight and shape. It is very important that you work with a therapist to set realistic expectations about weight loss and changes in your physical appearance before proceeding with surgery.

On the other hand, surgery does lead to very real changes in physical appearance in most cases. Learning to adjust to being seen differently, and usually more positively, can also be challenging. So, although you may never reach some "ideal," you are likely to change your appearance enough that you will have to address new issues, such as more social interaction, dating opportunities, and an increased energy for sports. It may seem that this will be easy to manage, but in fact, it is also stressful, and a therapist can help you examine your response to these "positive" changes as well.

For Teens

As a teenager, you are experiencing some of the biggest changes in your brain and in your emotional, social, and family life that you will ever undergo. Certain brain circuits are adapting to accommodate more efficient and abstract thinking. This means that you will be able to think through and evaluate problems in a more adult manner with each passing year. It appears that this process is one that continues well into the early twenties; what this means is that your analytical and decision-making ability is still incomplete in the teen years. Practically, this means that the process of making life-changing decisions, such as undergoing bariatric surgery, should be done with parental advice. Although this may not seem altogether reasonable to you, parental consent is required by law.

Not only is your reasoning ability being developed, but the way you deal with emotions is also changing. Those changing brain circuits and new levels of hormones in your body mean your emotional world may at times feel both exhilarating, and, at other times, confusing. Further, because you can think more about things, you are more aware of your feelings and their implications. Combined, these factors can give the impression that you are moody and changeable. The positive side of this is that you can be hopeful where others may be less enthusiastic. In terms of weight loss surgery, it may mean you will need to reign in your enthusiasm somewhat to tolerate the rather lengthy period of assessment.

Although one's social life changes during adolescence, if you are like many adolescents who suffer from obesity, your social life may not have changed as much as you wish it had. You might feel left behind because of your appearance, your physical limitations, or your own feelings of shame about your weight. You might have avoided flirting or dating because of this as well. As a result you may have high hopes about weight loss surgery's ability to change your social life. Although surgery may well change a great deal about your social life, you will still face the same challenges that most teenagers face—friends that don't meet your expectations, disappointments in dating, and limitations on your physical abilities.

You have probably noticed that you are trying to be more independent from your parents. Dealing with obesity and being evaluated for weight loss surgery may seem a step backward (or at least not a step forward). On the one hand, you want more privacy and more respect for your ability to make decisions using your growing intellectual, emotional, and physical independence, but at the same time you need your parents to agree with your decisions, support you in them, and provide ongoing support for you as you recover and start a new routine of caring for yourself. It will take patience on your part to work with your parents, but they can be your best supporters in this process. Certainly, problems with your parents should be a theme in your work with the therapist who is supporting you through this process.

Issues to Consider and Discuss With Your Therapist

Given the seriousness and the complexity of your decision to have weight loss surgery, you should take some time to work through the following list of discussion-provoking issues with a therapist (Readiness for Weight Loss Surgery form). Following your thoughtful analysis of all these issues, you will be in a good position to complete

Readiness for Weight Loss Surgery

Weight and Medical Status

_____

_____

_____

_____

Dieting and Exercise History

_____

_____

_____

_____

Binge Eating and Purging

_____

_____

_____

Emotional Issues

_____

_____

_____

(*continued*)

Trauma

_____

_____

_____

Alcohol and Substance Abuse or Dependence

_____

_____

_____

Social Support

_____

_____

_____

Commitment to Lifestyle Change

_____

_____

_____

Realistic Expectations

_____

_____

_____

the "double" costs-and-benefits analysis included below, where you will have a chance to examine the costs and benefits of both undergoing a weight loss surgery procedure and delaying it. Remember, you can always reverse a decision to postpone surgery, but you can never reverse a surgery that has already happened.

Are You Ready for Weight Loss Surgery?

In each section of the Costs-and-Benefits Analysis form below, write down the reasons that you think you should or should not have weight loss surgery.

Costs-and-Benefits Analysis

Pros and Cons of Weight Loss Surgery

Moving Forward With Surgery

PROS	*CONS*
_____	_____
_____	_____
_____	_____

Delaying Surgery for Now

PROS	*CONS*
_____	_____
_____	_____
_____	_____

Emotional and Interpersonal Readiness

Emotional and interpersonal readiness presents another set of issues to consider seriously before surgery. This means that you should begin to think about all that the surgery means to you in relation to, for example, following through with something you've wanted to do for yourself for some time to improve your life, while simultaneously facing the potential for negative consequences that are always a potential with radical surgery. Many emotions can surface as you consider the surgery; for example, you might notice feelings of guilt that you are "allowing" yourself to have surgery when you're not sure you deserve it, or anger that you have unfairly had to experience a weight problem to the degree that surgery is required. You will likely experience both anxiety and sadness as you face what lies ahead for you; but you will probably also feel great enthusiasm and excitement about the outcome and your new life after radical weight loss.

All these feelings will be linked in some way to various aspects of your changing relationship with food, your body, your sense of yourself, and your relationships with other people. As you delve into all your emotions about the surgery, you will need to stay well aware of the dichotomous nature of many of these changes. For example, your relationship with food will change following surgery, for both good and bad. On the one hand, you will be forced by the procedure to adopt a more healthy relationship with food; on the other hand, this will involve a loss in that you will no longer have the option of overeating to soothe yourself in the face of difficult emotions or situations.

Another cause of mixed feelings might be the actual results, as opposed to the ideal physical changes that you anticipated. Obviously, weight loss and all that comes with it, such as improved health, mobility, and appearance, is your goal in following through with weight loss surgery, but you won't be able to predict what the new and thinner you will look or feel like, or how your body will hold up once you've lost a massive amount of weight. Yes, your clothing sizes will eventually decrease radically. But certain other results might disturb you; for example, you may have an accumulation of excess skin that doesn't shrink back after you lose weight, you might have a hernia or lose some of your hair, and you could simply feel disoriented in a body that you no longer recognize.

In addition to thinking through all the feelings that are likely to arise as you progress in your surgery, it is important to consider your strategies for communicating with your loved ones, friends, acquaintances, and others all that you want them to know about what you are and will be going through. You might focus this discussion within yourself by thinking through how to tell your loved ones and others about your expectations and fears about the surgery, including your concerns about a poor outcome or even death; and how they can help you before, during, and after the procedure (while also gently sharing with them your sense of what they might inadvertently do that would be harmful to your process).

The point here is not to be maudlin but rather to have you realistically assess what is happening inside you as it relates to your upcoming surgery so that you can decide what needs to be discussed with others. Taking the time to do this well in advance of the surgery makes it much more likely that you will have a clear and level head.

Exercises for Exploring Your Feelings About Surgery

This section provides exercises to help you thoroughly examine and write about your deepest thoughts and feelings about the weight loss surgery you are about to undergo. As you get closer to the date of surgery, you might notice that your thoughts and feelings change; thus it is important to keep an ongoing journal of where you are at in relation to your surgery.

Deservingness

The Why I Am Deserving of Weight Loss Surgery and How it Will Improve My Life form on page 35 provides an opportunity for you to write about why you deserve the surgery, what types of positive changes you are hoping the surgery will effect, and what you have been doing to care for yourself as you prepare for it.

Ambivalence

The exercise on page 36, My Concerns About Undergoing Weight Loss Surgery, might be more difficult. It returns to the idea of the mixed bag of feelings that often come with complicated terrain like radical surgery. Specifically, it addresses the "costs" aspect of the costs-and-benefits analysis you completed earlier. Here, it is important that you take time to think through and freely express in writing any and all of the fears, concerns, worries, or misgivings you might have about the surgery. Of course these will differ from person to person, but the list might include attention to some of the physical risks associated with undergoing any surgery, weight loss surgery in particular, including the risk of mortality; general worries about complications, physical discomfort, and difficulties with healing; or more "trivial" worries associated with being in the hospital, finances, time away from your usual activities, and the like. By the same token, it is also essential that you explore any issues of entitlement that you might have about the surgery and your recovery. Here, entitlement means assuming a somewhat grandiose attitude that denies the potential for adverse effects associated with the procedure or difficulty recovering from it. Although staying positive is obviously of the utmost importance, not blinding yourself to the potentially negative consequences of the surgery (see the section immediately below) is also essential. Without allowing for both the positive and the negative, you will not be prepared to take yourself and your self-care seriously at all stages of the surgical expe-

Why I Am Deserving of Weight Loss Surgery and How It Will Improve My Life

_____

_____

_____

_____

_____

_____

_____

_____

_____

_____

_____

_____

My Concerns About Undergoing Weight Loss Surgery

rience: preparation, initial recovery and healing, later recovery, and long-term maintenance of change.

A Changed Relationship With Food and Eating

The third exercise, My Relationship With Food and How It Will Change After Surgery, is found on page 38. It pertains to your relationship with food and eating and how these areas of your life will be affected by the surgery. Obviously, it is impossible to understand before surgery the extent to which your relationship with food will change after surgery. But clearly your relationship with food and eating will be profoundly and permanently changed (unless you have lap-band surgery, which is to some extent reversible). While individuals may become obese for different reasons—for example, due to a strong genetic predisposition and/or longstanding habits of over-eating combined with inactivity—for most, food likely has provided a significant source of emotional and physical gratification.

After surgery, your relationship with food will have to be more "deliberate," careful, and mechanical, at least until your new eating habits become second nature. Thus, despite the fact that the net effect of having weight loss surgery should be that your appetite decreases and you feel full more quickly, at first you will have to give considerable thought to the experience of eating to comply with your doctor's orders regarding the timing, contents, and portions of meals and fluid intake. This requirement makes one's relationship with food anything but spontaneous; one can no longer react—to emotions, hunger signals, cravings, or situational factors—by eating; whereas before the surgery, many obese people acknowledged that most of their eating was "in response to" some type of triggering agent that often had little to do with satisfying hunger or taking weight management into consideration.

Simply stated, food and eating can no longer be used "recreationally." There will probably be feelings of sadness, loss, frustra-

My Relationship With Food and How It Will Change
After Surgery

tion, or even anger in addition to a very strong need to fill the void that food once occupied in meeting so many of your needs. In thinking through the earlier section on the costs of undergoing the surgery, it is very important to devote special attention to how your relationship with food will change postoperatively and how this might affect you. The next exercise will help you focus on shifting your mind to activities that don't involve food but that can be at least somewhat pleasurable and gratifying (even if initially they are not as stimulating to you as food has been).

Alternative Pleasures Not Linked to Food

While the question, "What can you do instead of eat when you want to eat for reasons other than hunger?" may seem stupid or simplistic, it is important to spend some time examining your answer. Use the form on page 41 to explore this question. Many people who have been obese for years have allowed food and their weight to dominate their lives, such that other interests, hobbies, and relationships have receded. Take some time to consider a range of other emotionally gratifying or meaningful ways to spend your time and energy, so that you have a list of reasonable alternatives to eating that makes you feel interested in something, interesting, and engaged. Ideas that have worked for others include taking a warm bath or shower, gardening, going for a walk, calling a friend, looking up information on the Internet, watching TV or a movie, and going for a short drive. In addition, specific relaxation techniques can be helpful. Some of the standard relaxation strategies include deep-breathing exercises, progressive muscle relaxation, and using visual imagery. Instructions for using deep breathing exercises, progressive muscle relaxation, and visual imagery can be found below:

Deep-Breathing Instructions
1. Sit in a relaxed position.
2. Place your hands on your lower belly.

3. Breathe in deeply so that your belly expands with each breath.
4. Imagine that you are breathing in clean, pure, beautiful air.
5. When you breathe out, feel your belly contract, and picture yourself letting go of any stress or tension.

Progressive Muscle Relaxation

1. Starting with your lower legs, tense your feet for five seconds while breathing in, and then relax as you breathe out.
2. Follow this process with your calves, then your quadriceps, and then your thighs, tensing and then relaxing each muscle group separately, coordinating your breathing as described.
4. Now focus on your lower back, stomach, and pelvis in turn.
5. Move to your upper back, chest, and shoulders, again tensing each group for five seconds and then relaxing.
6. Do the same for your hands, and then your face.
7. Finally, breathe in and tense your entire body, and then relax, letting go of your breath and all your tension and stress.

Visualization Exercise

1. Imagine a scene in which you feel entirely relaxed (the scene might include lying on a beach, taking a walk outdoors, visiting a place that has special meaning to you, etc).
2. Think through all the details of the scene that enhance your feeling of relaxation. For example, in the case of the beach scene, you would think about the temperature, the feeling of the sun on your skin, the smells and sounds of the ocean or other body of water, birds flying overhead, and the color of the sky and the sun.
3. Revel in each of these details as they inspire you.
4. Make sure to insert yourself into the scene, and as you enjoy the calm associated with your image, observe that you are totally relaxed, safe, and at peace.

What I Will Do to Fill the Voids Without Eating

When Surgery Goes Badly:
Preparing for Unlikely Complications

Finally, as you have become more and more aware of the potential costs and benefits of the surgery, the issue of mortality has probably occurred to you. While the goal here is not to encourage you to dwell on worries about dying as the result of surgery, it is important that you come to terms with the possibility, no matter how remote, and make peace with yourself regarding your decision about the surgery and other aspects of your life, and make peace with the significant others who are affected by all that happens in your life, including potentially losing you. The way you get in touch with your feelings about death will be quite personal; there is no one way to approach preparing yourself and others for the remote possibility that you could die as the result of what is in most cases an elective surgical procedure. Nevertheless, you should take some time to really think through these issues. For example, you might consider writing a letter to your significant others that says all you would want to say to them if this were your last chance to say it. You might even want to incorporate some of what you wrote about your decision to have the surgery, so that they fully understand the entirety of your experience.

Given the likelihood that all will go well with your surgery, it is of the utmost importance to plan and to prepare others to support you in the most helpful ways possible. For example, you might request that certain family members or friends drive you to the hospital, stay while you are undergoing the procedure, and be there when you wake up afterward. You might ask others to help stock your kitchen with the foods and beverages you will need during the first few weeks after surgery. Still others might be called upon to visit you while you are at home, to drive you to follow-up visits and other appointments or activities, or to provide emotional assistance in the form of "a shoulder to cry on" if you need that when you become anxious or worried before or after the procedure. In lining up support, your ability to communicate your emotional state and your needs to your significant others is essential. Unless you tell them, they will not know that, in addition to feeling very excited about your upcoming surgery, you are also anxious, worried, or struggling with guilt about whether or not you deserve it. If you don't let people know what you are experiencing and what you need, they can't possibly respond.

For Teens

Obviously, if you are a teenager, your parents will be highly involved in all aspects of the presurgical and surgical processes. You will not be on your own. You will want to make sure that they understand the work you have done presurgically with your therapists and with yourself to make you (and them) confident that you can succeed. Parents always worry about their children. However, undergoing the preparation for surgery with you will enable them to be a great resource for you. Try to identify how your parents can be specifically helpful to you—tell them who you want with you when you go to the operating room, what you want waiting in the recovery room, and how much and when you want others (friends and relatives) to know about the surgery and how you're doing afterward. Your parents will likely be in charge of making sure all the immediate discharge medications are ready when you go home.

Chapter 3   *Weight Loss Surgery Procedures: What You Need to Know*

Common Weight Loss Surgery Procedures

Currently, there are a few popular procedures. Some are only restrictive in nature, meaning that a new, smaller stomach "pouch" is created and the exit of food from the stomach is limited (slowed gastric emptying), and some are also malabsorptive, meaning that the surgery changes how food is absorbed as it leaves the stomach and enters the small intestine, usually because part of the small intestine is re-routed or removed. Some surgeries lead to more rapid weight loss and more complications. Some procedures are "open," meaning that they require a larger abdominal incision; some can be laparoscopically performed, with the surgeon—at some centers assisted by a robot—operating via a camera that goes through a small incision; and some surgeries can be performed either way. The surgeries that are the best studied, most accepted, and most commonly performed are the laparoscopic adjustable-silicone gastric banding (lap-band)

and the roux-en-Y gastric bypass (RYGB). Some surgeons still perform a biliopancreatic diversion, although many consider this surgery to be on the decline because of the higher rates of complications and technical difficulties. See Table 3.1 for a more detailed description of these and other less commonly performed procedures.

Risks and Benefits

Each surgery has its own risks and benefits. Table 3.2 describes common complications and nutritional deficiencies reported with each surgery. Unfortunately, the quality of the research done on weight loss surgery has been suboptimal, although it has improved in recent years. In 2005 the Cochrane group published an updated review and analysis of all the literature to date on weight loss surgery, attempting to identify the effects of surgery for morbid obesity on medical illness, weight, and quality of life. This analysis identified only 26 studies out of 3,223 published references as being of high enough quality to use in their report, and most of these 26 studies still contained much bias, according to the reviewers. This does not mean that the publications were invalid but simply that they are preliminary and often do not compare different surgical approaches to each other or to other weight loss methods, did not use appropriate research procedures to "randomize" patients (necessary for comparing different approaches), and/or did not follow patients for a long enough period of time (at least 12 months) to be able to detect long-term effects. What it does mean is that despite a lot of research on obesity surgery, there are many things that doctors still do not know and need to learn, and you should consider this fact. Like any other significant medical procedure, there are known risks, and in this field, there may be additional risks that are not yet understood by the medical community. Make sure to thoroughly consider this when making your decision, and to discuss it with your physicians, as you

Table 3.1 Surgical Procedures

Restrictive Procedures	Vertical Banded Gastroplasty (VBG)	In this procedure, the stomach is divided divided by a line of staples to produce a much smaller gastric pouch that holds only about an ounce. The outlet of the new pouch is similarly small, about 10–12 mm in diameter. This outlet empties into a section of stomach that then empties, as before, into the small intestine. The surgeon usually reinforces the outlet with mesh or Gore-Tex. The VBG may be performed with an open incision or laparoscopically.
	Siliastic-Ring Vertical Gastroplasty	A variant of the gastroplasty described above. Here, the stomach is again divided by a row of staples to produce a small gastric pouch. In this procedure, the new, smaller outlet of the new gastric pouch is reinforced by a silicone band to produce a narrow exit into the stomach, as detailed above.
	Laparoscopic Adjustable Silicone Gastric Banding (LASGB or lap-band)	This surgery, known as the lapband, was was approved by the U.S. Food and Drug Administration in 2001. It is performed only laparoscopically, as its name indicates. Here, a new gastric pouch is formed with staples, as with the gastroplasty, but the band surrounding the outlet from the new pouch into the stomach is adjustable because the band is connected to a reservoir that is implanted under the skin. The surgeon can inject saline into the reservoir, or remove it from the reservoir, in an outpatient setting to tighten or loosen the band, thereby adjusting the size of the gastric outlet.

| Restrictive Malabsorptive | Roux-en-Y Gastric Bypass (RYGB) | The RYGB is the most commonly performed procedure. It involves creating a small (⅓–1 oz) gastric pouch by either separating or stapling the stomach. This pouch drains via a narrow passageway to the middle part of the small intestine, the jejunum, bypassing the duodenum, through which food normally traverses before arriving at the jejunum. The older portion of stomach goes unused and maintains its normal connection to the duodenum and the first half of the jejunum. This end of the jejunum is then attached to a "new" small intestine created by the procedure above. This forms the "Y" referred to in the name of the procedure. This redirection of the small intestine is a malabsorptive featurecomplementing the restrictive feature that is the smaller gastric pouch. RYGB may be performed with an open incision or laparoscopically. |
| | Biliopancreatic Diversion (BPD) | This surgery is considered more technically difficult and so is less commonly performed. It involves a gastrectomy that is considered "subtotal," meaning it leaves a much larger gastric pouch compared with the options described above. The small intestine is divided at the level of the ileum (the third and final portion of the small intestine), then the ileum is connected directly to this midsize gastric pouch. The remaining part of the small intestine is then also attached to the ileum. This procedure thereby bypasses part of the stomach and the entire duodenum and jejunum, leaving only a small section of small intestine for absorption. |

(*continued*)

Table 3.1 (*continued*)

Biliopancreatic Diversion with Duodenal Switch (BPDDS)	BPDDS is a variation of BPD. It preserves the first portion of the duodenum, the first section of the small intestine.
Jejunoileal bypass	This surgery bypasses large portions of the small intestine; it is no longer recommended in the United States and Europe because of the high rate of complications and mortality.

are the only person who can assess how much risk you are comfortable with.

Similarly, think twice about trusting a physician who treats the idea of obesity surgery lightly, as if it is no big deal or your only option, as this is not a reasonable conclusion to draw from what we know. Surgery might be an appropriate option for you, especially if you have endured years of poor health, poor quality of life, low self-esteem, and social stigmatization because of extreme obesity and have made multiple unsuccessful attempts to lose weight using other methods. A good, experienced surgeon will be the first to admit that there are risks from the surgery and these should be considered along with the benefits when determining whether bariatric surgery is right for you.

First, it is important to remember that this is a surgical procedure, done under general anesthesia, and therefore certainly carries a risk of complications, including possible death. The rate of each risk varies with the age, health, and weight of the patient and with the type of surgery. Morbidly obese patients are considered "high-risk" patients for surgery, because a higher dose of anesthesia is used, the surgery is more difficult to perform, and their overall health is often poor, increasing the likelihood of possible complications. However, data from the International Bariatric Surgery Registry—a registry of more than 10,000 patients—reveals a 30-day mortality rate of 0.3%. Other published studies have shown 30-day mortality rates of anywhere from 0.2% to 1.9%. One study of Medicare beneficiaries (who are thought to have potentially poorer overall health) showed a 30-day mortality of 2.0% and a one-year mortality rate of 4.6%. Mortality rates are higher in older patients, especially those older than 65 at the time of surgery.

The experience of your surgeon has a major effect on both mortality rates and rates of re-hospitalization in the years following surgery. Studies show a direct correlation between the surgeon's caseload (how many bariatric surgeries he or she performs regularly, which usually also reflects his or her experience level), and lower mortality and re-hospitalization rates. You should choose a doctor who is board certified in surgery and who is a member of the American Society for Bariatric Surgery.

Which Surgery Could Be Right for Me?

Again, the literature comparing different types of surgery has not approached a degree of sophistication that permits one to make firm recommendations about which surgery is "right" for which person. The mortality risks of the surgeries have not been well compared, for example. For this reason, physicians are still uncertain as to the true differences among all the surgeries. However, we can discuss some general trends in the few studies that make such comparisons.

In general, research suggests that restrictive surgeries are associated with less weight loss over time, fewer side effects like dumping syndrome (see Table 3.2, page 52), fewer long-term nutritional deficiencies, more revisions, and a higher possibility of weight re-gain when compared with bypass operations. However, a few studies do not show a major difference in weight loss among procedures. The lap-band is an option that has enjoyed success in other countries. Compared with vertical banded gastroplasty (VBG), it is associated with more gradual but overall greater weight loss over time, fewer weight-loss related complications, and higher patient satisfaction. One study showed more late complications and revisions after lap-band procedures than after gastroplasty. Initially, the lap-band requires frequent follow-up visits to adjust the band's width. These restrictive operations do not alter the absorption of food from the intestine; they change only how much food the stomach can hold and how quickly it exits the gastric pouch.

In most studies, restrictive-malabsorptive procedures see more rapid weight loss and a greater improvement in quality of life, but they can have more complications, both in the short and long terms. The RYGB is the most commonly performed of these and is considered the gold standard by many surgeons. All restrictive-malabsorptive procedures affect how food is absorbed in the intestines, thus making it more likely that nutritional deficiencies will develop and requiring the patient to take vitamins and other supplements for the rest of his or her life to help prevent such problems. Some procedures, like the biliopancreatic diversion (BPD) and biliopancreatic diversion with duodenal switch (BPDDS), cause more malabsorption than others, like the RYGB. Some studies have also reported more surgical complications following bypass surgery than VBG or lap-band. However, by altering the anatomy of the small intestines, these surgeries change the hormones in the intestines that affect hunger and fullness cues. Many patients report not feeling hungry after surgery, and one study reported a reduction in the urge to binge eat after malabsorptive procedures. Researchers are working to understand more about these changes and what they mean for long-term health. These changes may explain why some diabetes in patients resolves immediately after surgery, even before any true weight loss has occurred. Many studies have shown a dramatic improvement postoperatively in other conditions as well, especially obstructive sleep apnea, hypertension, obesity hypoventilation syndrome, and gastric reflux. Again, such changes are not universal after malabsorptive procedures, and it is very important to balance the risks against the benefits, as these procedures certainly involve long-term diet and lifestyle changes to prevent serious complications.

While BPD and BPDDS can lead to more weight loss, these procedures involve the most malabsorption and thus have the highest rate of malnutrition-related complications. They (especially BPDDS) are considered the most technically demanding of weight loss surgeries and should be undertaken only by a surgeon who has a good track record with this particular method. The stomach size is not reduced to the same extent as in the other surgeries, and many patients can therefore tolerate larger amounts of food in the years after surgery; also BPDDS avoids most incidences of dumping syndrome. However, more complications are reported with these methods, and all these factors should be considered when deciding which surgery is right for you.

A final consideration is whether to have your procedure performed via an open incision or via a laparoscope. As for bypass and adjustable banding procedures, open and laparoscopic surgeries get similar weight loss and quality of life scores over time, but complications are not uncommon with either type. Occasionally, laparoscopic surgery has to be converted to open surgery, and this rate differs in different studies. Laparoscopic surgery can take longer, but the studies are inconsistent in this regard; some research has shown a longer hospital stay with open procedures. VBG results in similar weight loss, fewer wound problems and scars, higher patient satisfaction. Many surgeons now perform only laparoscopic procedures (at some centers robot-assisted) whenever possible, as it seems there are fewer surgical complications with them.

Table 3.2 Reported Complications of Bariatric Surgery

Complication	Description
Atelectasis and pneumonia	Atelectasis is a potential complication of any surgery, is worsened by obesity, and refers to small portions of the lungs that can collapse after surgery, often due either to general anesthesia or to the immobility associated with abdominal surgeries postoperatively. If untreated, it can lead to pneumonia, which can significantly delay recovery and is a more serious condition. Patients are therefore asked to get up and walk as soon as possible after surgery, often the first day.
Blood clots (DVTs and pulmonary embolus)	Deep vein thromboses frequently develop in obese, immobilized patients. Surgery on an obese patient can increase the likelihood of their occurrence. Pulmonary emboli occur when clots in the deep veins of the leg break off and travel to the lung, causing potentially life-threatening problems. The surgeon may prescribe blood thinners, special stockings, and walking soon after surgery to help prevent clots.
Cardiac problems	These are more common in patients with histories of heart problems, high cholesterol, and diabetes, and can range from myocardial infarction to sudden cardiac death. These conditions are known to occur more frequently in obese patients regardless of surgery. Sudden cardiac death has also been reported in patients with rapid weight loss from high-protein liquid diets and may be more likely to occur if weight loss is rapid, significant, and not carefully medically monitored.
Death	Mortality risk can vary depending on the type of procedure and surgeon. Make sure to discuss this risk with your surgeon.
Diarrhea and dumping syndrome	Malabsorptive procedures (especially BPD and BPDDS) are associated with diarrhea in the months after surgery. This is usually because of the inability of the body to absorb fat. Dumping syndrome is caused

Complication	Description
	by food leaving the stomach and entering the small intestine too fast and can cause diarrhea, cramps, dizziness, sweating, and rapid heart rates. Dumping syndrome is more likely to occur with sugars, high-fat foods, and simple carbohydrates.
Expansion of the stomach pouch	Expansion can occur idiosyncratically or because of excess food intake over time. Some doctors believe the intake of carbonated beverages contributes to expansion. The larger the stomach pouch becomes and the more closely it begins to resemble a normal-sized stomach, the closer the person can come to near-normal food intake and possible weight gain.
Gallstones	Many patients develop gallstones after weight loss surgery, often requiring the removal of the gall bladder. This complication occurs because of a combination of rapid weight loss and alterations in bile acid secretion due to anatomic changes after surgery. Studies have shown more men than women developing this complication.
Incisional hernia	This happens when the intestine or abdominal fat "pokes" through the stitches after surgery. Sometimes hernias cause no symptoms, but occasionally a part of intestine can become trapped in the hernia, requiring emergency surgery. Often they need to be surgically repaired, but if they are minor, this can be done after most weight loss has occurred.
Intestinal obstruction	Sometimes bands of scar tissue can form in the abdomen and "trap" parts of the intestine, causing a blockage that prevents the passage of food and liquid. Blockages can also result from an "internal hernia," which occurs when the intestine slips through suture lines within the abdominal cavity. All obstructions need to be repaired surgically.

(*continued*)

Table 3.2 (*continued*)

Complication	Description
Intolerance to certain foods and liquid	Sometimes patients report difficulty with certain foods that are healthy and desirable in their diet, such as vegetables and other high-fiber foods or large volumes of liquids, which are often required after surgery to keep hydrated. Intolerance can make dietary management difficult, and it needs to be closely followed until the problem is surmounted. Intolerance usually results because the stomach pouch has been reduced so much by surgery, and there is an increased dietary need for protein and liquid.
Loose or sagging skin	Depending on the amount of weight lost, the age of the patient, the length of time he or she has been obese, and the quality of the person's skin, plastic surgery to remove excess skin might be recommended, particularly if there are skin irritations or infections resulting from overhanging folds of skin, such as the *pannus,* the "apron" of skin that folds over the abdomen after weight loss.
Malnutrition	This is more common after malabsorptive procedures and can cause various symptoms, including a weakened heart, hair loss, dry skin, nutrient deficiencies, metabolic problems, electrolyte changes, ankle swelling, and muscle loss. Malnutrition can be avoided by carefully adhering to the prescribed diet and by taking all supplements.
Nutrient deficiencies	See Table 3.3.
Strictures	These narrowings of the gastrointestinal tract can occur after surgery and are usually related to excessive scarring. They tend to occur at levels of the intestine or stomach that have been altered by the surgery. Symptoms of stricture are an inability to tolerate solids or liquids and excessive vomiting. The strictures can often be "dilated," or widened, by passing a

Complication	Description
	balloon through a small camera into the GI tract (endoscopy).
Surgical complications associated with any intraabdominal surgery	Blood transfusion, allergic reactions, risk of anesthesia, blood loss, accidental organ injury, bladder infection (from catheter placed during anesthesia)
Surgical leak	Leaks occur when stitches or staple lines closing off the stomach or small intestine break open. Breaks allow digestive fluids normally contained in the intestine to leak into the abdomen and can cause infections and other problems. Breaks require immediate surgical repair.
Ulcer	In bypass and malabsorptive procedures, part of the intestine is cut and a different portion is reattached to the stomach. This part of the small intestine is more vulnerable to "marginal ulcers," ulcers resulting from the strong stomach acid that that portion of intestine is not accustomed to. Often, these ulcers can be treated with medicines.
Wound infections	Infection is more common in obese patients, as their abdominal wall is thicker. Up to 10% of open abdominal weight loss surgeries result in infections. Wound infections occur less commonly after laparoscopic procedures. Good wound care postoperatively can help prevent infection.

After Surgery: What Do I Do? What Do I Eat?

Most experienced bariatric surgeons work with a team of professionals to help manage patients both pre- and postoperatively. Usually, the team will consist of the surgeon, a physician, a dietician, an exercise therapist, and a social worker or other mental health professional. This team works together to help patients manage their body and mind as they notice rapid changes over the first year after surgery; all members of the team are essential to long-term success. The recommendations the team gives you about postoperative management will depend on your overall health status and the type of surgery performed. However, here we will discuss general recommendations that pertain to most patients after weight loss surgery.

Diet

Right after surgery, your calories will be reduced significantly, usually to fewer than 1,000 per day, divided among five or more small meals and snacks. Patients are prescribed only liquids initially and are slowly advanced to pureed foods; they can eat solid foods later but must adjust gradually. After gastroplasty or RYGB, the gastric pouch is very small and can manage only a small amount of liquid or food at a time. Patients undergoing BPD or BPDDS surgeries can manage slightly more food, as their stomachs are not as small postoperatively, although they are at higher risk of malabsorption-related nutritional deficiencies (see Table 3.3, page 58).

A high-protein diet is important for at least the first six months following surgery because weight loss is rapid, and both fat and muscle stores are lost. It is very important to ingest at least 60 grams of protein per day to preserve muscle stores and prevent protein-calorie malnutrition. Often, patients are advised to drink large quantities of liquids. Sometimes patients need to drink liquids separately from eating solids to allow the maximum protein intake at meals. All patients need to take certain supplements and vitamins after surgery—usually at least a multivitamin, calcium, iron, and a B-vitamin supplement. To prevent dumping syndrome after malabsorptive surgeries, it is important to avoid simple carbohydrates, high-fat foods, and sugars. Carbonated beverages are discouraged after all procedures because they cause uncomfortable bloating that can that can affect the size of the gastric pouch.

Exercise

You will be directed to exercise immediately after surgery. Most comprehensive teams include an exercise therapist and a structured exercise plan. This is important both to prevent complications related to immobility (partial lung collapse, deep vein thromboses, etc.) and to maximize weight loss while minimizing loss of muscle stores. It is also an important lifestyle change that elevates mood, minimizes the chance of weight re-gain, and improves lifelong health.

Overall Health

Your doctors should be monitoring your health closely. Frequent visits to the doctors and surgeons that help coordinate your care is often necessary immediately following surgery, with many physical exams, weight checks, and labs. Usually, the focus is on adjusting your treatment to address any chronic medical illnesses you might have (you may be able to reduce certain medications quickly after surgery), looking for surgical complications, and monitoring you for nutritional deficiencies (see Table 3.3). Your team will also be monitoring you for depression, anxiety, or other mental health changes you might experience as a result of changes in your body, lifestyle, and physical health. The changes you will undergo are big and will take some time to get used to. Some patients have more difficulty than others.

Table 3.3   Potential Postsurgical Nutritional Deficiencies

Type of Deficiency	Description	Treatment/Prevention
Calcium	Fatigue, muscle twitches/tingling, heart palpitations, poor bone health and osteoporosis	Calcium citrate is preferred preparation; should take 1200–1500 mg daily; may be adjusted if dietary intake is good
Electrolyte: potassium, magnesium, phosphorus	Can lead to heart arrhythmias and other muscle problems; described in varying frequencies after weight loss surgery	Immediate supplementation if prescribed
Folate	Occurs less frequently than B12 deficiency but can also cause anemia, psychiatric changes	Multivitamin; folic acid supplement may be prescribed
Iron	Anemia, fatigue, paleness; more common in menstruating women	Daily multivitamin with iron and possibly iron supplement
Protein-calorie malnutrition	A severe form of macronutrient deficiency that can result in muscle loss, low albumin levels, swelling in the ankles, and when severe, heart problems or even death	Attention to optimal protein intake before and especially after surgery
Vitamin A	Vision changes, night blindness, dry eyes, dry skin	A multivitamin and dietary changes usually suffice to prevent
Vitamin B1 (thiamine)	Usually manifests as headaches, irritability, and fatigue. Can cause Beriberi (cardiovascular changes,	Immediate treatment with thiamine; may need treatment in a hospital

Type of Deficiency	Description	Treatment/Prevention
	neurologic/sensory changes), Wernicke's encephalopathy (clumsy gait, nystagmus, or rapidly vacillating eye movements, and sometimes memory changes); in rare cases leads to neurological damage and/or death	
Vitamin B6	Skin inflammation, sore tongue, depression, confusion, and convulsions, anemia	A multivitamin and dietary changes usually suffice to prevent
Vitamin B12 (cobalamin)	Occurs in >30% of patients after malabsorptive procedures, including RYGB. Can cause fatigue, anemia, numbness, tingling, confusion, mental slowing	Vitamin B12 supplement in daily or monthly injections
Vitamin D	Muscle weakness, bone pain, poor bone health, rickets, osteoporosis	Multivitamin, dietary intake of dairy if tolerated; may need ergocalciferol or other vitamin D preparation
Vitamin E	Neurological changes, heart problems, confusion, weakness, blindness	A multivitamin and dietary changes usually suffice to prevent
Vitamin K	Bleeding difficulties	A multivitamin and dietary changes usually suffice to prevent

Nutritional Deficiencies

Unfortunately, postsurgery vitamin and nutrient intake and deficiencies have not been well studied after weight loss surgery. Severe protein malnutrition is uncommon with the VBG, lap-band, and RYGB but does occur after the BPD and BPDDS, both of which cause more malabsorption and thus can result in protein malnutrition. Vitamin and mineral deficiencies can occur after the RYGB, BPD, BPDDS, and any surgery with a malabsorptive component; they have occasionally been reported after VBG as well. Multiple types of deficiencies, including of vitamins A, D, E, K, B1, B6, B12, folate, and iron, have been described. The most common of these are discussed in Table 3.3 in more detail.

Chapter 4 *Navigating the System*

Taking the Plunge: Required Preoperative Evaluations and Consultations

Once you decide definitively to proceed with weight loss surgery, you will face a number of challenges.

The fundamental ones are:

- Obtaining referrals from your primary care physician (PCP) and any other physicians involved in your care who are recommending and making a case for the necessity of your weight loss surgery.

- Getting your insurance to cover the costs of the procedure, which can be considerable (see later section on the costs of surgery). Typically, this involves your PCP's recommending the surgery as a necessary treatment for certain medical problems associated with your obesity and documenting the facts of your weight problem, for example, BMI, weight and dieting history, and concomitant medical issues.

- Researching and locating a skilled and experienced surgeon connected to a well-respected hospital with a comprehensive weight loss surgery program. The surgeon needs to be appropriate for you (e.g., someone that you feel comfortable with who is also willing to work with you and your insurance and is covered by your particular insurance plan).
- Scheduling and following through with the additional consultations required by your surgeon and his or her team. These will likely involve a consultation with an internist, a gastroenterologist, a registered dietician or nutritionist, a mental health professional such as a psychiatrist or clinical psychologist, and possibly a cardiologist and/or additional physicians, depending on your particular physical health issues.

How to Get Started Once You Know What to Do

The following section should help you navigate the system better as you prepare for your surgery. It should also help you anticipate and work through any emotions, such as anxiety, that you might feel as you plan for and follow through with these professional consultations.

Obtaining a Referral From Your Primary Care Physician

If you've been struggling with obesity for some time, it is likely that you've discussed the matter with your physician at some point, and that he or she probably told you that you should "lose some weight" to improve your health, whether or not serious health problems were ever diagnosed. Your doctor is in a good position to help you with respect to "authorizing" weight loss surgery as the appropriate next step in your weight loss process and thereby supporting you in getting your insurance company to cover the surgery as a medically necessary one. (In the event that you are in prime health despite your problem with obesity, and/or if you are on the "border" of what is considered clinical obesity, your insurance company might not cover the surgery.) No matter what your health status, your first step needs to be getting in touch with your primary care doctor, if you already have one, or finding one that you can work with, if you don't.

Your primary care physician will ultimately be responsible for documenting your request for a referral for weight loss surgery and providing information about your current and past obesity-related health problems, your attempts to diet and the outcome of those diets, and any important tests or examinations that should be done before surgery to clarify additional health issues that may have surfaced. Typically, the PCP, with your written permission, will write a letter to both your surgery team and your insurance company to support your need for weight loss surgery.

In most cases, the next step will be to contact your insurance company about their policy for covering this type of surgery. It may take you some time to get enough information from your carrier to determine whether or not the surgery might be covered. For that reason, as soon as you begin to consider a weight loss surgery procedure, you should document all the steps you take to get the surgery covered. For example, write down all interactions you've had with your physicians and other medical personnel in your pursuit of the surgery, and record details of any current or past dieting efforts. All your discussions with your insurance company, whether by phone, e-mail, letter, or in person should also be recorded. This documentation may be needed at later stages for any number of reasons (e.g., to "prove" that various statements were made by the insurance company, to attest to your current and past efforts to resolve your weight problem nonsurgically, and to ascertain your motivation, persistence, insight, good judgment, and clarity in thinking as you continue to pursue surgery as the solution to your weight problem).

If you are encouraged by your insurance company to think that the surgery might be covered, that is a good sign. However, a guarantee of coverage takes time and will ultimately be made only after your PCP and the other professionals with whom you consult during preoperative planning and "diagnosis" regarding the necessity and suitability of surgery in your particular case have provided all the required information. Your insurer's determination that surgery is necessary will also be affected by its view the appropriateness of a particular type of surgery (e.g., lap-band versus duodenal switch) to your specific needs. The importance of knowing in advance your surgical options and the suitability of these, given your particular needs, cannot be overemphasized.

Handling Doctor Visit–Related Anxiety

It is common to experience anxiety when meeting with your surgeon or other health professionals involved in evaluating you for gastric bypass surgery. The following sections highlight strategies to reduce medical visit–related anxiety.

If you are someone who becomes anxious, particularly when meeting with individuals you consider authorities or experts—such as your surgeon and the other professionals with whom you might consult, it is important that you get a handle on those feelings before the appointments so that they do not get in the way of your asking the questions you need to ask and providing the information the surgeon needs from you. It is helpful to adopt a "problem-solving in advance" mindset: envision the issues that might "trip you up" during the meeting and take steps to address them in advance. You should then imagine how you want the session to go. You might, for example, sit with your eyes closed for five or ten minutes and visualize the interaction, stopping to calm yourself with deep breathing or helpful thoughts such as "It will be OK. I will feel competent, deserving of professional attention, and justified in any questions I might want to ask during my appointment."

You should also write down all the questions that you want to have answered during the session. Remember to bring the list with you! In some cases it might be a good idea to role-play the meeting by having a friend or significant other be the surgeon, with you playing yourself, and then reverse the roles. Also, it can be very empowering to bring a significant, trusted other (spouse, family member, friend) to the appointment with you so that you have "two pairs of ears" listening for information and taking in other aspects of the interaction. Finally, in your therapy sessions you will be discussing all the thoughts and feelings you may be having that are associated with the professional consultations that are required in the evaluation phase.

Choosing a Surgeon and What to Expect From Him or Her

After meeting with your PCP and getting the go-ahead from him or her, you will need to locate a surgeon with whom you want to work, who is available to work with you, and who may be covered by your health insurance. Ask your PCP for referrals, speak to others in your area who have already undergone weight loss surgery or are considering it, look up resources on the Internet using such search terms as "weight loss surgery," or request the names of qualified surgeons in your area from national associations, such as an association of weight loss surgeons or other obesity specialists. Once you identify potential surgeons, research their credentials. For example, you will want to know the number of weight loss surgery procedures they have done, whether or not they are board certified, whether or not they have ever been sued for negligence or malpractice, and how they have been evaluated by other patients in terms of surgical skill, bedside manner, and the like.

Once you select a surgeon and schedule a meeting with him or her, you should be prepared for any of the following. The meeting with your surgeon might take place before *or* after you see the various other health professionals involved in the preoperative screening process, depending on the policies of the particular center you are working with. Either way, it is likely you will feel some anxiety before meeting the surgeon—this is normal under the circumstances. The following information can help you counter that anxiety and feel more comfortable and relaxed when you do meet your surgeon for the first time.

Your appointment will probably take place in some kind of clinic or doctor's office. Your surgeon will likely ask questions about your current physical and mental health and your health history, your successful and unsuccessful attempts at dieting, and your exercise habits. He or she will try to get some sense of your rationale for considering surgery at this time and attempt to determine your current state of mind to ascertain whether or not you are psychologically ready to undergo the procedure. In considering your state of mind, he or she may ask you specific questions about your mental health and drug and alcohol use and general questions about your lifestyle, including habits such as smoking and exercise. The surgeon will also ask about your eating habits including any particular eating problems such as binge eating, eating late at night, drinking excessive amounts of soda or other fluids, and so on. Much of this information will be supplemented with records that the surgeon has obtained from your PCP (such as a letter referring you to the weight loss surgery program, lab results, and/or your entire medical record) and the other health professionals that you may have consulted before meeting with your surgeon.

For example, if you've already met with the dietician, your surgeon will review his or her notes and any food logs you completed.

Similarly, if you have already formally completed the psychological evaluation with your current therapist or another mental health professional, the surgeon will read that person's report before your appointment and discuss the implications of the report's conclusions with you. Also, depending on the particular weight loss surgery program and surgeon you are working with, you might be asked during or before the session to fill out a number of questionnaires to be discussed with you later. These might ask about your mental and physical health; your past and present eating, dieting, and exercise habits; your strategies for coping with stress; and the extent to which you use food to cope. Your surgeon might also recommend any number of diagnostic tests before you are accepted into the surgical program or invited to schedule your surgery. These tests could be related to the functioning of your gastrointestinal system, respiration, sleep, blood, or emotional functioning. The surgeon might also wish to know more about your social support network. Each center and each surgeon will have a different preoperative process and will likely recommend a slightly different array of tests (with the internal medicine and gastroenterology consult, the psychological evaluation, and the nutritional assessment included in most, if not all, cases).

Based on the dietician's and mental health professional's findings, the surgeon might also recommend that you postpone surgery until certain issues are addressed (for example, binge eating, severe depression, alcohol abuse, recent trauma) or even that you forgo surgery altogether. To address any issues that might be ameliorated to an extent that would enable you to have the surgery at a later date, the surgeon or other members of the evaluation team might recommend that you participate in regularly scheduled psychotherapy sessions, undertake group therapy, or perhaps take medication (such as an antidepressant). In addition, the dietician's recommendations will be taken into consideration by the surgeon. These might reflect the presence of a specific eating habit or problem (for example, binge eating or eating habits likely to impede weight loss that need to be addressed before surgery) or a more general knowledge deficit when it comes to food issues, dieting, and weight control.

In addition to the mental health professional and possibly the dietician, your surgeon will likely also attempt to assess your understanding of the nature of the surgery, the risks and probable benefits, and the lifelong changes in eating and activity patterns that you will need to make to truly benefit from the surgery. Many surgeons are now recommending a weight loss before surgery of about 10% of your baseline weight. The reasons for this vary but might include making the surgery safer (by reducing your size and improving your health), improving your "candidacy" for laparoscopic rather than "open" surgery, and, to some extent, testing both your motivation and your ability to comply with a behavior modification plan that dictates moderation in eating and exercise (if possible). It is also quite common for surgeons to recommend that patients join a weight loss surgery support group well before their surgery date. A support group will expose you to additional knowledge regarding all aspects of weight loss surgery from start to finish. Patients are usually encouraged to participate in this type of group regularly (e.g., monthly) for some time after surgery. Such participation helps one gather useful information about both the positive and negative outcomes of weight loss surgery and enhances one's support network to include those with firsthand knowledge of the entire surgical process; group members are better able to maintain objectivity than even very supportive significant others.

Your Session With the Evaluating Psychologist

Just as you were anxious about meeting with your surgeon, you might be anxious about your session with the mental health professional (referred to here as the psychologist) who will formally evaluate you. To quell your anxiety, we will review the rationale for this session and describe the structure of a typical meeting. Remember that the evaluating psychologist and the other professionals consulting with you (including your therapist) before your surgery are aligned in their mission to help you make the best decision about your upcoming surgery. *Everyone is on your side and has your best interests in mind.*

The purpose of the psychological evaluation is to determine from a mental health perspective if you are a good match for weight loss surgery in the near term. Determining your basic fit and readiness for surgery are the primary questions this evaluation strives to answer, and the interview will reflect this; the questions may be more or less complex, depending on your situation.

The mechanics of the session will likely be similar to the meeting with your surgeon. Although the psychologist might be slightly more casually dressed, you will probably meet in a professional office similar to the surgeon's, whether located in a clinic, office building, or house. The session might last as little as 45 minutes or more than an hour, depending on the setting, the psychologist with whom you are meeting, and your particular issues. Depending on the center and individual practitioner, you might be asked to fill out a number of questionnaires (before or during the session) pertaining to your mental health, including your past and present emotional state, the stability of your mood over time, any past or current treatment for emotional issues, and your coping style, support system, and expectations for weight loss surgery. These questionnaires may be discussed with you during the session or at a later date.

Typically, the psychological interview is one-on-one. In most cases significant others are not included, in order to allow you maximum privacy to share your personal story and details of your struggle with weight, food, and other issues. Although in some cases your loved ones might be invited to join the psychological evaluation session later, it is best to expect that most of the time you will be sitting alone with the mental health professional interviewing you.

You will emerge from this session with new information and a number of recommendations. For example, you may be given a time-line for scheduling the procedure based on your needs and the scheduling issues at your particular surgery center. You might also be given specific suggestions for addressing certain issues and making certain lifestyle changes before surgery. These could include a recommendation to undertake specific behavior modification strategies related to changing your eating and activity patterns to help with weight loss. Or, you may be encouraged to engage in a psychological or medical intervention to address emotions or behaviors (e.g., "talk therapy"— the kind of therapy you should already be engaged in with your therapist, or, alternatively, treatment with psychotropic medications). On the other hand, you might be strongly encouraged to delay the surgery, to cancel it altogether, or to hasten the process and undergo surgery as soon as possible.

In any case, if you recognize that the psychologist *is on your side*—there to help you make the best decision regarding your surgery—your experience will be a good one. With this attitude in mind, there should be no obstacles whatsoever to your providing as frank and honest a portrayal of your current life situation as you can. This will include responses to the psychologist's questions about your thoughts, feelings, and behaviors related to eating, exercise, and self-care, including your strategies for coping with stress and other strong emotions, whether these strategies are known to be beneficial to you (such as doing physical exercise to work off stress) or somewhat harmful (e.g., using drugs, alcohol, overeating, purging, or any other compulsive or dangerous behavior). You will be asked by the psychologist about the current state of your weight problem and your history of struggling with it, including when your weight problem first developed and what efforts, if any, you have made to lose weight, and how successful they were. While in most cases, it will be the dietician or nutritionist, and not the psychologist, who will obtain very detailed food records from you, possibly covering a recent one- to three-day period, the psychologist might also question you about your daily schedule, possibly asking how you spend your time most days and seeking more information about your eating patterns. This will help him or her determine the extent to which binge eating and/or other particular and problematic eating habits might be primary causes of your weight problem. Current and past treatments to address these issues will be reviewed. The psychologist might also ask your permission to speak with mental health professionals with whom you have worked or are working.

The psychologist will also ask "why now"; that is, how have you come to consider weight loss surgery as an option, and what has been happening in your life to prompt the decision to pursue surgery at this point? The degree to which you understand the various surgical options, how the surgery is done, how and why it works, your role in contributing to a positive outcome, and the associated risks and potential benefits will also be explored. Obviously, it will be in your best interest to research the surgery as much as possible before you forge ahead with any of the evaluation sessions. And clearly your knowledge base will be conveyed in the consultation sessions, showing that you are proceeding in a responsible fashion and exercising sound judgment and thoroughness in determining if weight loss surgery is right for you, and in what form and when.

Following the session, the psychologist will, in most cases, document the visit by writing a report that addresses all the areas noted above, along with a summary that includes his or her impressions and recommendations. The recommendations will likely include suggestions for improving the preparation process (e.g., working with a physical therapist to develop an exercise plan and participating regularly in a weight loss surgery support group). In cases in which there are obvious impediments to proceeding with surgery, the psychologist might recommend that you seek treatment for a mental health, substance abuse, or other problem *before* scheduling a surgery. (Perhaps it is such a recommendation that prompted you to start therapy with your current therapist.) Typically, the findings of this evaluation are communicated in writing to the surgical team. Generally, the psychologist will not say that the surgery should or should not be undertaken but will provide commentary that allows the surgical team to concur—or not—with a suggestion for you to proceed with, delay, or forgo the procedure.

Most psychologists will be direct with patients about the report they will send to the surgical team and sometimes also to the PCP. Most psychologists do not release these types of reports directly to patients, although they must provide them if requested. It is most productive for the patient and evaluating psychologist to review the findings together, so that the report, including all questions and concerns, can be interpreted for the patient and its contents not taken out of context or misunderstood. Such a process minimizes miscommunications. If during or after your session you are worried about what the psychologist is thinking or which pieces of information that you shared will be included in the report, it is best to simply ask! It is important that you are as up front as possible with the psychologist about any worries or anxieties that you might have after this session so that these can be addressed and resolved.

It is important to keep in mind that the best approach to the psychological evaluation is to be honest. For example, portraying yourself more positively in the hopes of then being deemed an appropriate surgical candidate is never in your best interest when this contradicts reality. Remember, the psychologist ultimately has your best interests in mind in his or her attempts to evaluate your psychological state and elements of lifestyle that might render you unsuitable for immediate surgery. The psychologist is there to help you make the best decision, not to thwart your progress. Keep in mind that by concealing problems, you might come across as desperate to create a positive impression and, consequently, as someone who cannot be trusted to present a realistic picture of issues and problems that may lurk beneath the surface, even if they are only mild or moderate in nature. This falsely positive presentation is the surest way to signal a mental health professional that you are deceitful or dishonest in presenting yourself. Lying will therefore only hurt you; once a lie is detected, the mental health professional will have trouble trusting your responses to other questions during the interview. Furthermore, your tendency toward dishonesty will most certainly be noted in the psychological report to be reviewed by the other professionals with whom you will be working. Certainly, their ability to trust what you say about yourself will be compromised once dishonesty is revealed.

Your Meeting With the Dietician

The session with the dietician (who may also be called a "nutritionist," depending on his or her degree and credentialing) will likely be similar in many ways to your meetings with some of the other professionals. You will probably spend up to an hour with the dietician, and you may be encouraged to schedule one or more follow-up sessions. In most cases, the session will be held in a private office. The dietician may or may not be connected to the medical center at which you will be having your surgery. In some instances, the weight loss surgery program will allow you to work with a dietician you already know (e.g., if you have been consulting with someone on issues such as weight management, diabetes control, or any other concerns). In other instances, the program might require that you work with a dietician specifically connected to their program, whose expertise in evaluating patients before weight loss surgery is already well established. Usually, the person you meet with will be a registered dietician, which means that he or she has passed certain licensure requirements in the state in which you live.

In some cases, before meeting with the dietician, you will be asked to keep records of your eating patterns for a period of three days or more. (Forms for recording your daily food intake and the amount and type of daily physical activity you undertake are included later in this chapter.) You will also be asked to clarify whether or not you are currently making efforts to diet, and if so, how these have altered your typical eating patterns. Also, depending on the particular weight loss surgery center and the individual practitioner with whom you are working, you might be asked to fill out a number of questionnaires, either before or during the session, that pertain to past and present eating habits and attitudes. Usually, these will be reviewed at least briefly during the session, as the dietician strives to understand as much as he or she can about your relationship to food and eating. For example, the dietician will determine whether you generally maintain a schedule of regular meals or snacks, "graze" frequently on small amounts of food throughout the day, or go for long periods without eating anything at all and then overeat or binge, in a context not typically associated with overeating for others. Other questions might focus on your tendencies to eat large quantities of food late at night or even after you've gone to sleep, or to drink large amounts of fluids, such as sodas or juices. The dietician will also ask you questions about current or past purging—that is, using strategies such as vomiting or overuse of laxatives in an attempt eliminate excess food.

Based on your dietary recall and the information you share during the interview, the dietician will assess your current and past caloric intake and will note whether or not you are adhering to your "typical" eating patterns or are dieting. He or she will estimate the number of calories that you should be consuming to lose weight steadily before surgery—if that has been recommended—; likewise, the dietician will estimate how many calories you should consume after surgery and will advise you on one or more dietary strategies to help you restrict calorie intake and lose weight. In addition, your current and past relationship with exercise will be examined. Depending on your level of fitness, individual health concerns, physical limitations, familiarity and comfort with various types of exercise, and the advice of your primary care physician, the dietician might talk with you about various exercise options likely to facilitate your weight loss.

During the session, the dietician will also be sizing up your general knowledge base about nutrition issues. You will probably be asked about your understanding of what calories are and how calories contribute to changes in weight, the calorie counts of some of your favorite foods, and your sense of the calorie ranges you would need to stay within to progressively lose weight. Your knowledge of other matters of nutrition may also be assessed, such as your understanding of the health contributions of the major nutrient groups: protein, fat, and carbohydrates, the ways in which these are incorporated into a balanced diet, and their relative contributions to hunger and fullness.

If you have been asked by the surgical team to lose weight before surgery, some of the session will focus on helping you create a presurgery weight loss plan to achieve that goal; in many instances, doctors recommend a weight loss of 10% before surgery, but this varies greatly from case to case, and some surgical candidates may be discouraged from losing any weight at all. For example, some centers might ask you to participate in research studying the impact of losing or not losing weight before surgery; some patients may therefore be asked not to lose weight before the procedure. In making recommendations, the dietician will consider your past successful dieting efforts (e.g., following structured, commercial plans such as Weight Watchers, Optifastv or other liquid protein diets, Jenny Craig, or Atkins; or following your own strategy of counting calories and increasing your physical exercise) and the central components of each, to emphasize strategies that are appropriate and that proved successful for you (at least in the short term). Also, aspects of your lifestyle that are likely to have a significant impact on your efforts to lose weight will be taken into account, for example, your food preferences, exposure to high-risk eating situations, proximity to problem foods, level of physical activity, stress level, and degree of mental fortitude and physical resilience that can be applied to the challenging and often frustrating terrain of dieting.

The discussion will also include a detailed evaluation of your current physical activity patterns and some recommendations, subject to approval by your PCP, for beginning a mild exercise regimen or adding to your current routine, if your current activity is seen as not strenuous enough to facilitate weight loss, reconditioning of your body, or both. For example, occasionally patients are encouraged to begin walking 10–30 minutes a day, up to a few times a week, or to participate in some form of water exercise before surgery. The latter can be helpful in that it is a low-impact activity that is easier on the body than many other forms of exercise that can be painful for obese persons already struggling with lower-body or other joint or extremity pain. Although some weight loss surgery programs will include or suggest that you consult with a physical therapist or even a personal trainer with expertise in working with obese clients, remember that, no matter what, you should always consult with your PCP about any and all exercise before embarking on a new regimen, particularly if you are excessively obese and/or have very serious physical problems that make even short, slow walks of several yards difficult.

A portion of your session with the dietician will focus on helping you learn how to eat after surgery. You will probably be given various handouts containing guidelines. These will most likely include a description of the various postoperative "phases," each of which dictates a slightly different eating strategy. For example, in the first few days and weeks after surgery, most programs emphasize a high-protein liquid diet of very small portions consumed at regular, specified intervals (e.g., 2–4 ounces every 2 hours). Many programs encourage patients to add pureed and then soft food over the next few weeks, and eventually more solid foods. All these suggestions include very clear guidelines about portion control, emphasizing, for example, the importance of initially eating servings that are no more than two to four ounces, and then slowly and steadily increasing the size of servings over time to no more than 6–8 ounces at a time, maximum. Also, there will probably be suggestions about which foods you should avoid for periods ranging from weeks to a year; you will likely be asked to permanently eliminate some foods from your diet. The specific nature of these suggestions will vary, depending on the type of weight loss surgery you will be having and the philosophy and approach of the dietician with whom you are working. But the list will likely include meat, sweets, alcohol, carbonated beverages, certain bread products, and possibly other foods that are hard to digest after weight loss surgery.

During the nutrition evaluation, it is likely that you will also have a chance to discuss certain postsurgery eating trends and patterns that have been observed for other patients. For example, following weight loss surgery, many patients find that their food preferences, tolerances, and intolerances change quite radically. Some postoperative patients might report great tolerance for a wide variety of foods, including healthy fare such as fruits and vegetables and less-desirable foods such as sweets. On the other hand, some might report difficulty with vegetables or other foods considered desirable from a health and weight maintenance standpoint.

Ultimately, to make sense of the array of inputs and suggestions about your food intake postoperatively, it might be best to think about comparing, contrasting, and integrating all that you've heard and read. For example, you will get both verbal and written recommendations from your dietician and your surgeon, and you might also come across certain materials on the Internet and through discussions in your weight loss surgery support group. Obviously, should there be any discrepancies, you will want to discuss these with your surgeon. But it is important to keep in mind that in many cases there is more than one right way to eat following surgery. So, rather than adopting a perfectionistic, black-and-white attitude about postoperative eating, it is best to anticipate shades of gray: you will need to assess your individual needs, preferences, and judgments about what is best for you and incorporate all of this data into your decisions about food. Remember, it is probably extremes in your thinking about food (e.g., "one slipup and I've blown it") that contributed to your weight and eating problem in the first place.

The culmination of the nutrition evaluation will be handled similarly to how the sessions with the other professionals have been handled. For example, at the conclusion of your session with the dietician, he or she will summarize the session and provide an evaluation of the strengths and weaknesses of your eating patterns, your knowledge base about food and dieting, and your readiness for weight loss surgery. Any written materials that were part of the evaluation will be included in the report, which will be sent to the surgical team and possibly also to your PCP. Should you have any questions about what the dietician will say in the report, or what he or she is thinking—about your eating habits or any other aspect of your weight issue—you should ask. Remember: don't be afraid to raise questions with any of the consultants.

A Comprehensive Checklist

The following checklist can help you keep track of where you are in terms of these numerous preoperative requirements. Your diary or journal will also prove useful to help you keep track of the process. Following the checklist are discussion questions and exercises to help you get in touch with several of the crucial issues related to your surgery.

Have you:

1. Found a program you like?
2. Identified a surgeon with whom you are comfortable, who has accepted you as a patient and offered the weight loss procedure that you want?

3. Been referred to this program and surgeon by your primary care physician (PCP)?

4. Determined if your insurance will cover the surgery, or found other financing?

5. Met with a program-endorsed:
   a. Dietician?
   b. Mental Health Professional?
   c. Internist?
   d. Gastroenterologist?

6. Followed through with the professionals' recommendations:
   a. To keep records such as food and exercise logs?
   b. To start to lose weight and/or exercise, if this is required?
   c. To begin to recondition yourself in preparation for surgery (e.g., improve eating patterns, nutrition, activity level), if weight loss is not required?
   d. To start counseling, therapy, or medication treatment for a mood issue?
   e. To begin any other necessary medication or treatment (such Continuous Positive Airway Pressure [CPAP] for sleep apnea)?
   f. To make follow-up visits with the dietician, if this was recommended?

7. Begun to think at a deeper level about the experience of undergoing a radical surgery, to emotionally prepare for the surgery, and to discuss these issues with significant others or other members of your support network? This work should include:
   a. Getting in touch with your feelings about surgery, including reviewing the costs and benefits of the procedure;
   b. Examining your feelings of guilt, anxiety, deservingness, and entitlement and how these might affect your behaviors postoperatively;
   c. Thinking about the ways in which your relationship with food

will change after the surgery and trying to identify strategies for filling the voids left by this change by incorporating gratifying and meaningful activities not related to food;

d. Looking at the positive and negative aspects of your relationships with others to prepare an interpersonal stance that will allow you to hold on to healthy attitudes about your decision to undergo weight loss surgery no matter what others say.

e. Planning in advance to share at least some of the above, including your anxious thoughts and feelings about any aspect of the surgery (including an untoward outcome such as death), with your significant others so that they can know in advance what you feel, what you need, and how they can help.

Home Exercises to Help You Prepare for Surgery

- Create a presurgery journal, if you have not already done so.
- Read and review the description of the professional consultation meetings.
- Decide upon a set of anxiety-management and relaxation tools to calm you before, during, and after these sessions.
- Complete and review the checklist in this chapter.

Chapter 5

What to Expect After Surgery

This chapter discusses what to expect immediately after your surgery and in the following few days and weeks. It will remind you of the importance of following the recommendations of your surgical team regarding your dietary intake, the amount of rest and physical activity you will need, and the necessity of being patient, using various supports, normalizing frustrations, and so on, in the short term.

Once you have undergone your surgery, you deserve to give yourself a big congratulations and pat on the back for following through on your goal—an undertaking that was extensive in terms of mental, physical, financial, social, and logistical challenges. You deserve to be commended for persevering and accomplishing what you set your mind to.

Hopefully, all will go well with your procedure. There are several steps you can take prior to your surgery. Before undergoing your surgery, it can be particularly helpful to identify those who will be able to care for you at various stages before and after the operation. For example, you should have a complete list of people who will be available for you, and the specific tasks that you would like each of them to perform (if they agree). You will want to know well in advance who will drive you to the hospital, who will stay while the procedure is completed, and who will be there to visit you in the first hours and days after the procedure (assuming there are no complications). Think about what, if anything, you would like each person to bring when they come to visit you and in what capacity they can be "on call" for you, should you have an unanticipated need.

You will also want to know who will be there in the days and weeks after the procedure when you're recovering at home. For example, you will want to know who will prepare the simple meals that you need and bring them to you if you are having trouble getting around. At some point before your surgery, you will also want to make a detailed list of all the food and other supplies you will need so that you or one of the members of your support team can purchase these necessities during the initial postoperative period. Also, you may need special first aid supplies on hand to treat your healing incision wounds. You might be prescribed certain vitamins or other medications that need to be picked up and prepared a certain way (crushed, halved, or softened). In addition, it will be important that you restart all medications that you were using before the surgery if your physicians recommend that you continue them. Particularly important is restarting any medication to regulate mood. Knowing before surgery how you and others will keep track of all these necessities is essential so that nothing comes as a complete surprise to anyone.

Finally, you will be required to make a number of postoperative follow-up visits scheduled at various intervals after your surgery, depending on the practices of the surgical center, the type of procedure that was done, the initial surgical outcome, and your particular health needs. Since it will be weeks (depending on the exact nature of the surgery) before you can drive, you will need to arrange for members of your support team to drive you to these visits. It goes without saying that no follow-up visit should be missed, as it is at these meetings that your surgeon and members of the team fully assess your progress. After they make their assessments, your team may make suggestions, adjustments, or interventions.

It is at these visits that you will be able to get consistent and reliable data about what is happening with your weight, relative to others who have undergone the same procedure. While you might be one of the few who has a scale at home able to accurately measure your weight both before and after surgery, the scales at physicians' offices are more accurate than typical home scales.

The Postsurgery Journal (pages 84–86) and checklist (page 87) that follow can help you organize the above information, and you should of course feel free to add as many people and tasks to your list as you want.

Assuming that the first few days at home have gone well, you might feel quite relieved, if not euphoric, that you have made it through this crucial stage of healing. Once you become aware that the first few days have passed uneventfully, it's possible that you will start to worry about the surgery, or you may start to hastily develop future plans. For example, you might become somewhat anxious about some of your body's reactions to the surgery and/or some of the bodily changes you observe (such as continued pain at the site of the wound(s) or changes in your bathroom habits). Alternatively, your mind may already have jumped to what the next few stages of healing, recovery, and adjustment will be like. Some people may even feel an initial, somewhat catastrophic, reaction of "what have I done to myself?"—a type of buyer's remorse. This reaction reflects anxiety about the unpredictability of what's in store and how things will progress and evolve over the next few days, weeks, and months.

While some level of anxiety might help motivate someone to keep them on track after weight loss surgery, too much anxiety can shut a person down and so prevent them from caring for themselves correctly after surgery. For example, entertaining highly anxious thoughts, also known as "catastrophizing," might cause a person to lose sight of the positive aspects of their decision to undergo surgery and of all the improvements to come as they lose weight. Instead, they

Postsurgery Journal

Postsurgery Journal (*continued*)

Weight Loss Surgery Support, Supplies, and Tasks List

Supplies List

1. _____

2. _____

3. _____

4. _____

5. _____

6. _____

7. _____

8. _____

9. _____

10. _____

Support Team Member	*Assignments for Him or Her*
1. _____	_____
2. _____	_____
3. _____	_____
4. _____	_____
5. _____	_____
6. _____	_____
7. _____	_____
8. _____	_____
9. _____	_____
10. _____	_____

may be aware only of pain and exhaustion, stiffness and soreness, and other unpleasant sensations accompanying most radical surgeries. Or they may choose to focus on some of the specific, slightly disorienting changes this surgery caused their bodies, such as having a distinctly different experience of appetite that requires very extreme changes in eating habits. These imposed physical and behavioral modifications might initially feel scary and permanent, and thoughts like "it will always be like this" might occur, along with worries such as "what if the surgery doesn't work and I don't lose weight?" or, "what if it wasn't worth it?"

Managing Anxious Thoughts After Surgery

If you start experiencing anxious thoughts after your surgery, it is very important that you stare them in the face, embrace them, and then sensibly "massage" and transform them into thoughts that are less worrisome and more constructive. You will know when appropriate and healthy thoughts are on board because these will be oriented toward keeping you in an optimistic frame of mind. These positive thoughts help you stay on the right track regarding a successful recovery from your surgery. They also help keep you focused on your commitment to learning to relate to food and your body in a new and healthier way.

A technique you can use to combat your negative, anxious thoughts after surgery is outlined below. Consult Figure 5.1 for an example of how this works, and use the Changing Your Negative Thoughts Worksheet (page 90) to perform the exercise yourself.

How to Change Your Negative Thoughts
1. Write out the core problem thought in simple terms.
2. List the objective evidence (not just your feelings but actual data) to support the problem thought.
3. Do the same for the objective evidence that argues against the problem thought.

Figure 5.1 Example of Problem-Solving Exercise

Problem Thought:

Everyone is watching me because they think that I weigh too much to be eating so much at this meal.

Supportive Evidence:

1. I see more glances coming my way from other people.
2. My daughter said, "Mom, do you really need that?" when I reached for a piece of pie.
3. When my brother saw me he said, "Wow, it looks like you've gained weight, and I thought you were dieting. Are you going to be eating with us?"

Disconfirming Evidence:

1. It was kind of a free-for-all at the table—everyone was interacting with everyone about food and other topics, too.
2. People in our family always comment on others' weight and what others are eating; this is just how it is in our family.
3. Some other family members are overweight, too.
4. I know that I have been watching my weight and that I had deemed this a special meal that I could indulge at a little bit. Given that, I was doing pretty well at this dinner.

Reasoned, Evidenced-Based Conclusion (that will lead to positive behavior):

People may have been watching me (or maybe not), but it really doesn't matter what they say or think about my weight and eating because I know that I was doing my best with food at this special meal and that it didn't ruin my diet. So the last thing I want to do is overeat because of them and my interpretations of what they were thinking. I will make an even firmer commitment to eat healthfully, for myself, not because of anyone else.

Changing Your Negative Thoughts Worksheet

Problem Thought:

_____

_____

_____

Supportive Evidence:

_____

_____

_____

_____

Disconfirming Evidence:

_____

_____

_____

_____

Reasoned, Evidenced-Based Conclusion (that will lead to positive behavior):

_____

_____

_____

4. Come up with a reasoned conclusion based on the evidence to guide you to appropriate and healthy behavior.

At such times of anxiety, when you may be second-guessing your decision about the surgery, it is very important to figure out what other options are available to help ease your anxiety. You may wish to use the worksheet below to create a list of pleasurable, alternative activities in which you can partake that don't involve food or eating. Obviously, you will be somewhat limited in the early stages of recovery as to what you can and can't do, but you should create a short list that includes simple, relaxing, and sedentary activities such

Pleasurable, Alternative Activities

1. _____

2. _____

3. _____

4. _____

5. _____

6. _____

7. _____

8. _____

9. _____

10. _____

as reading, watching TV, looking up information on the Internet, chatting with a friend, and so on. It is very important to overcome any signs of anxiety in this early postoperative stage because anxiety can cause you to act out—that is, engage in a behavior that is ultimately not in your best interest given your desire to heal adequately after surgery and get on with the business of serious weight loss.

After you have had at least a few weeks to adjust to the changes associated with your surgery, you should have a sense of how you are coming along in terms of following through with the dietary recommendations appropriate to your recovery stage, feeling comfortable with those changes in eating, and losing weight at an appropriate rate. At your regular follow-up meetings with your physician, he or she should provide feedback on your progress (including documentation of your continuing weight loss) and encouragement to stay on the right track. These messages should correct any misperceptions that you may have been struggling with regarding how things "should" be going as opposed to how you are actually doing and should address any problem behaviors that you've been exhibiting. Within the first few weeks and months after your surgery much of your focus will be on ensuring that you are handling your food and liquid intake correctly, losing weight, healing from the wounds of surgery, and generally staying positive and optimistic about all you've been through and are hoping for.

Mind and Mood

At some point in the first few months after surgery, you might be ready to shift your focus from your body and the physical changes you are going through to your mind and your mood. You might even deliberately begin a process of asking yourself how you're *really feeling*—in an emotional sense—to get in touch with this deeper or subtler layer of perception that you might have overlooked while busy keeping your body on track and healthy after surgery. Although there are no established research statistics that specify the exact percentage of people who might develop significant mood problems (such as depression or anxiety) at some point after weight loss surgery, there is always the possibility that a mood issue will develop. It is logical to assume that this may be particularly true for those individuals for whom mood issues were a moderate or serious problem in the past.

On the other hand, those individuals for whom mood issues were not problematic before surgery might nevertheless be affected by mood problems after. Again, without actual data to support it, this vulnerability might be more pronounced in those who relied on food to a great degree, in the form of binge eating or other types of compulsive eating, to regulate their mood, or relied on other substances or alcohol for the same effect. In any case, given the very dramatic physical changes following the radical weight loss made possible by weight loss surgery, even previously nondepressed and nondistressed individuals might begin to feel some unpleasant mood changes postoperatively. Be prepared for this.

Depression

In terms of sizing up a depressed mood, if you were falling into a depression, you would most likely experience at least some of the following symptoms: a feeling of sadness, a sense of pessimism that is inconsistent with the positive decisions and changes you have made, tearfulness, distractibility, difficulty getting up to greet the day, difficulty performing your usual activities (at least those appropriate in your recovery stage), and in the worst cases, suicidal thoughts or plans. Clearly, if you were thinking of suicide, you would likely already be painfully aware of your depressed mood and would not need to do any structured form of self-inquiry about your mood state. (On the other hand, certain individuals can become quite skilled at hiding from themselves and others—or denying—negative mood states such as depression.) In any case, if the low mood were this severe, it would likely be "announcing itself" to you and your therapist rather than lying dormant and hidden. You and your therapist would next try to understand all the circumstances contributing to your mood. You would then discuss how to work through these problems (both from the biological perspective, possibly seeking a psychiatrist's or other medical doctor's opinion, and also from the psychosocial perspective). It is most important to talk to the team of professionals already involved in your care, including your surgeon and primary care physician. You should also consider disclosing your difficulties to your trusted significant others so that they know what is happening. Discuss with your therapist the possibility of increasing the frequency of your sessions together. Becoming more involved in some type of a support group or other ongoing, structured activity that typically has made you feel better will also help. At some point, your spouse, partner, or other family members might be asked to join you for one or more therapy sessions or to take part in family or couples therapy with you (separate from the work you are doing individually).

Once you have let at least one, and hopefully a few, of the doctors you are working with in on the fact that you are struggling with your mood, you will find that they have numerous suggestions for helping with your depression (in addition to all the work you are doing with your therapist in therapy sessions). For example, they might recommend that you start on an antidepressant medication, switch medications if you are already taking one, increase your dosage, or restart a medication you may have discontinued but that was helpful before.

Anxiety

As with depression, you will likely be the first to know if you are experiencing anxiety due to feeling "stressed," "under strain," or "fearful," and if you are having persistent intrusive and ongoing worries. The presence of moderate or serious anxiety would warrant your consulting with the members of your professional team, as well as your therapist, just to make sure that those caring for you and advising you about your medical issues are aware of what is going on; disclosing to significant others what you are going through; and thinking through, together with your consultants the viability of medication, additional psychotherapeutic interventions (e.g., an anxiety-management group), and so on. Although to date there has been only limited clinical and research data available to support this impression, it appears that serious anxiety postoperatively is more likely to occur in those with a history of anxiety or other difficulties in mood regulation. Postoperative patients may be left feeling particularly uncomfortable because they can no longer use unproductive solutions like overeating, binge eating, or substance use or abuse to escape difficult, anxious feelings. The key is to work with your therapist to identify the best solutions for conquering your negative thoughts and feelings.

Problem Eating

Obviously, eating potentially presents problems after weight loss surgery. Ideally, after your surgery you will be following the program (in terms of all the eating suggestions) in full, for example, eating (and drinking) as recommended at the appropriate times and in the appropriate amounts, no more, no less. In the best case, following the program will result in your having no difficulties or problems. Unfortunately, even when a person is doing his or her best to follow the program to the letter, there might still be inadvertent or involuntary eating difficulties of one type or another. For example, one side effect of weight loss surgery is occasional vomiting or other gastric upsets after eating certain foods or, in rare instances, after eating anything. Although such difficulties are infrequent, some people may experience vomiting, diarrhea, or other problems that could cause dehydration in the short term or even some level of malnutrition over the long term because the body is not regularly absorbing enough nutrients.

There are also obvious and noteworthy physical consequences of repeated vomiting (or diarrhea for that matter), including soreness or sensitivity when swallowing or when using the bathroom. With time, there is a potential psychological effect; for example, the person who is vomiting or "dumping" might begin to fear eating because of the possibility of vomiting or having diarrhea again. This problem can develop into a full-blown food phobia that might resemble classic anorexia nervosa to some degree. The affected person is likely to deny hunger or appetite out of fear of the potential physical consequences. Clearly, if any of this is happening to you, it is imperative to address this problem as quickly as possible. You need to stay vigilant about your own eating patterns and habits and about the thoughts and feelings that eating conjures. Keeping regular food logs in which you document your habits can be quite useful for both you and your therapist as you try to fully understand your eating behaviors and associated attitudes and emotions. Also, it can be helpful to listen to your significant others' feedback based on their observations of your eating habits, even though you might initially bristle at like what feels like criticism. Whereas others' *constant* intrusion in a situation like this is obviously not desirable, when it comes to eating patterns, weight loss, self-care, and mood states (including anxiety and depression) those around you might sometimes see more clearly than you can.

Binge Eating

Another problem can be overeating or "binge-eating" episodes, which, after surgery, should obviously occur on a smaller scale than they did before. A pattern of overeating can develop slowly and insidiously or might appear all of a sudden, as if out of nowhere. Based on clinical impressions, it appears that people who had problematic binge-eating habits before surgery are at greater risk for redeveloping the problem after surgery (even if there was a considerable "binge-free" phase before the surgery) than those who had never binged. However, there is so far no research data proving this. In any case, there are a number of potential scenarios involving overeating that might develop. For example, in one person a craving for "just a little bit" of a certain type of food might trigger what ultimately becomes an overeating episode, at least from the standpoint of what is ideal in terms of recommended food content and quantity (even if this eating episode would have been considered perfectly acceptable before surgery). When the eating episode transitions from normal or acceptable to problematic, the person might begin to have negative thoughts, leading to even more overeating. This is what is known as catastrophic thinking. For example, after consuming a "non-optimal" food (or too much food of any kind), one might think, "Now I've gone and blown it! I am ruining my surgery and will never lose weight!" These thoughts would obviously be more likely to perpetuate problematic behaviors than would a more constructive thought such as, "OK, this was just a small indulgence and it would be best to quit now while I'm still ahead with no damage done."

Cravings

Another type of overeating or binging that might happen "out of the blue" involves developing a strong craving for a particular food. When you experience a craving, you may allow yourself a "treat" of some type and then end up feeling uncomfortably full. In your zeal to take in as much of the indulgence food that you want or "can" consume, you end up significantly overeating relative to the post–weight loss surgery recommendations. Some individuals in this instance might go on to experience "dumping syndrome" in response, partly depending on the amounts and types of foods ingested, which could result in stomach upset, sweating, trembling, diarrhea, and possibly vomiting. In this instance, as much as the "dumping syndrome" proves to be a negative reinforcer for overeating (maximizing the distress or negative consequence that results from overeating to the point that you would likely wish to avoid a repeat at all costs), some people may ultimately experience the "dump" as something akin to a "purge." When it is seen this way, as eliminating food from one's body, it enables the person to feel—even if illogically—that he or she has, in essence, rid the body of the excess food and calories and therefore "can do it again" if and when the urge strikes. (This is the same logic that keeps bulimic individuals tied to their habit of binge eating and purging.)

If this type of overeating has been a problem for you in the past, there may be a greater likelihood that you will develop such a pattern again, particularly if you have experienced mood issues related to all stages of the binge-and-purge cycle (for example, initial "pre-binge" anxiety, followed by a distracted euphoria during and immediately after eating, then panic as the reality of what you've consumed sets in, followed by discomfort as "awareness" returns and satiety registers, then more pre-purge panic, followed by calm, after purging). In all such instances of chronic and frequent (e.g., more than a few in a week or a few weeks) problematic eating, it is absolutely essential that you and your therapist focus on this problem as soon as possible.

In addition, you will want to discuss what is happening with your eating patterns (including any purge-like behaviors) with your primary care physician and surgeon. Their involvement is particularly important since they know what to look for in terms of potential physical damage or side effects that can stem from a combination of your surgery and this type of behavior, and they might also want to make suggestions about other staff you should consult (e.g., a gastroenterologist). It is also important that you and your therapist discuss having you undergo a psychiatric evaluation, in which your likelihood of benefiting from certain mood and appetite medications can be assessed and appropriate recommendations made. No matter the type of eating problem, always keep in mind that, in addition to your work with the medical professionals who are already part of your team (including your therapist) and any weight loss surgery support group meetings that you are already attending, you can always attend other types of group meetings (for example, Overeaters Anonymous) and expand your significant others' involvement in your care.

Alcohol and Drugs

Finally, one other cluster of problematic behavior patterns that can occur after any type of stressful life experience, such as radical surgery, is alcohol and drug abuse. People with predispositions to or family histories of this type of problem or who have themselves had substance-abuse problems even years before surgery (most programs require that patients are "clean and sober" for at least five years before weight loss surgery) are probably more at risk than those who have had no substance-abuse problems. However, as with the development of problematic eating behaviors, substance abuse can develop secondary to an untreated underlying mood disorder such as anxiety or depression. Clearly, quickly and appropriately treating mood-regulation problems after surgery decreases the probability that you will abuse food, drugs, or alcohol to manage your mood. However, if you do notice that substance-abuse problems are newly developing or resurfacing after your surgery, the same recommendations apply: you need to talk with your therapist about getting specific, expert substance-abuse treatment in addition to your therapy sessions as soon as possible. You should not, under any circumstances, concern yourself with thoughts that you have let down the members of your surgical or medical team or that you have broken the rules or will be getting in trouble. The simple fact of the matter is that you are in acute need of professional assistance if you are abusing or dependent upon any substance, and the sooner you are able to get appropriate treatment, the better off you will be.

Options for Seeking Help

In all instances involving mood, eating, and substance abuse issues, the problems are serious enough to require specific, expert, individual, professional assistance, and possibly some form of group therapy or support as well. Keep in mind, however, that *any* type of problematic feeling or behavior, no matter how mild, deserves attention and treatment, if that is what you want. Hopefully, your therapist met many of your treatment and support needs as you prepared for weight loss surgery. But at some point both you and your therapist might reevaluate the course of treatment and decide to make some changes, perhaps including working with someone else. Before making any changes, however, your therapist should help you address and challenge any notion that you might have about the importance of "keeping a stiff upper lip," as embodied in thoughts like, "unless my problem is severe and includes depression, anxiety, major eating issues, or substance abuse, I should not seek help." The reality is, even if you are doing amazingly well, or moderately well with the exception of a few minor problems, if you want extra help or assistance in the form of individual psychotherapy (which may or may not include a consultation for medications), couples counseling, or group interventions (e.g., Alcoholics Anonymous or Overeaters Anonymous) in addition to your weight loss surgery support group, or any other type of group forum, you should feel that you are entitled to seek it out. In terms of individual therapy, the chemistry or fit between you and your next therapist is important. There are several different schools of therapy that your current therapist can help you understand or that you might educate yourself about, just to know what your options are.

Cognitive Behavioral Therapy

Cognitive behavioral therapy (CBT)—which is likely the type of therapy you do with your current therapist—would basically address the types of thoughts you are having and the behaviors you are exhibiting relative to issues of your weight loss surgery, eating, weight, body shape, mood, self-esteem, cultural pressures to be thin, and other concerns. The sessions would likely be somewhat structured and driven by an agenda based on your and your therapist's ideas about appropriate goals for the stage of therapy that you are in. In CBT, you are often assigned homework at each session, so that in your between-session time you are encouraged to experiment with various new perspectives and behaviors you talked about in your sessions.

CBT Self-Help Manuals

This is a "short-hand form" of CBT therapy based on a written manual, used in conjunction with intermittent and brief (e.g., every other week for 20 minutes) therapy sessions to keep you focused on the tasks and issues presented in the book.

Interpersonal Therapy

Interpersonal therapy (IPT) is a less directive approach to treatment, although there is a clearly defined agenda that involves your talking about one or a few primary interpersonal problems integrally related to your eating issues and weight concerns. Examples of core interpersonal problems might be navigating a difficult transition, such as that associated with becoming a more assertive person; becoming thin for the first time ever or for the first time in a long time; frequently experiencing conflicts with other people; or working through unresolved grief. In the initial few sessions of IPT your therapist would encourage you to take some time to reflect on your entire social life, for example, the number, quality, and type of relationships you have now and have had in the past in an attempt to identify the core problem areas that are troubling you. In many cases, it turns out that these same problem areas have also been instrumental, to one degree or another, in triggering or perpetuating aspects of your disordered eating behavior and your weight problem.

Other Therapies

Many other types of therapy exist and are practiced in a form that could potentially be very helpful to someone with eating problems and weight concerns. These days, an extremely popular form of treatment is emotion-regulation therapy, in which an individual is taught a number of different strategies and tools to embrace, validate, and gradually change any excessive or unconstructive emotional reactions they may have in response to "charged" or stressful situations of one type or another. In addition, there are several nonspecific therapies that may offer support, encouragement, feedback, reality checks, and an opportunity for accountability that can be quite helpful. In every case, therapy is most helpful when it involves a combination of the right people at the right time and in the right circumstances. Given the significance of what you have been through, continuing with your current therapy or embarking upon an alternative approach with a new therapist might be something to strongly consider.

References

Agras, W. S., & Apple, R. F. (1997). *Overcoming eating disorders: A cognitive-behavioral treatment for binge-eating disorder, Client Workbook*. New York: Oxford University Press.

American Medical Association. (2003). *American Medical Association roadmaps for clinical practice: Assessment and management of adult obesity, a primer for physicians*. Chicago: American Medical Association.

American Psychiatric Association. (1994). *Diagnostic and statistical manual of mental disorders* (4th ed.). Washington, DC: American Psychiatric Association.

Arnow, B., Kenardy, J., & Agras, W. S. (1992). Binge eating among the obese: A descriptive study. *Journal of Behavioral Medicine, 15,* 155–170.

Bacon, L., Stern, J. S., Van Loan, M. D., & Keim, N. L. (2005). Size acceptance and intuitive eating improve health for obese, female chronic dieters. *Journal of the American Dietetic Association 105*(6), 929–936.

Bocchieri, L. E., Meana, M., & Fisher, B. L. (December, 2002). Perceived psychosocial outcomes of gastric bypass surgery: A qualitative study. *Obesity Surgery, 12*(6), 781–788.

Bruce, B., & Agras, W. S. (1992). Binge eating in females: A population-based investigation. *International Journal of Eating Disorders, 12,* 365–373.

Buchwald, H., Avidor, Y., Braunwald, E., Jensen, M., & Pories, W. (2004). Bariatric surgery: A systematic review and meta-analysis. *Journal of the American Medical Association, 292*(14), 1724–1737.

Buddeberg-Fischer, B., Klaghofer, R., Sigrist, S., & Buddeberg, C. (2004). Impact of psychosocial stress and symptoms on indication for bariatric surgery and outcome in morbidly obese patients. *Obesity Surgery, 14*(3), 361–369.

Burns, David D. (1990). *The feeling good handbook.* New York: Plume.

Cash, Thomas F. (1997). *The body image workbook: An 8-step program for learning to like your looks.* Oakland: New Harbinger.

Chobanian, A. V., Bakris, G. L., Black, H. R., Cushman, W. C., Green, L. A., Izzo, J. L., Jr., et al. Seventh report of the Joint National Committee on Prevention, Detection, Evaluation, and Treatment of High Blood Pressure. *Hypertension, 42*(6), 1206–1252.

Colquitt, J., Clegg, A. (2005). Surgery for morbid obesity. *The Cochrane Library Database,* No. 3, CD003641.

Dansinger, M. L., Gleason, J. A., Griffith, J. L., Selker, H. P., & Schaefer, E. J. (2005). Comparison of the Atkins, Ornish, Weight Watchers, and Zone diets for weight loss and heart disease risk reduction: A randomized trial. *Journal of the American Medical Association, 293*(1), 43–53.

Delin, C. R., Watts, J. M., & Bassett, D. L. (May, 1995). An exploration of the outcomes of gastric bypass surgery for morbid obesity: Patient characteristics and indices of success. *Obesity Surgery, 5*(2), 159–170.

Dement, William C., & Vaughan, C. (2000). The promise of sleep: A pioneer in sleep medicine explores the vital connection between health, happiness, and a good night's sleep. New York: Bantam Dell.

DiLillo, V., Siegfried, N. J., & Smith West, D. (2003). Incorporating motivational interviewing into behavioral obesity treatment. *Cognitive and Behavioral Practice, 10,* 120–130.

Expert Panel on Detection, Evaluation, and Treatment of High Blood Cholesterol in Adults. (2001). Executive summary of the third report of the National Cholesterol Education Program (NCEP) Expert Panel on Detection, Evaluation, and Treatment of High Blood Cholesterol in Adults. *Journal of the American Medical Association, 285*(19), 2486–2489.

Fairburn, C. (1995). *Overcoming binge eating.* New York: Guilford.

Greenberg, I., Perna, F., Kaplan, M., & Sullivan, M. A. (2005). Behavioral and psychological factors in the assessment and treatment of obesity surgery patients. *Obesity Research, 13,* 244–249.

Grilo, C. M., Masheb, R. M., Brody, M., Burke-Martindale, C. H., & Rothschild, B. S. (2005). Binge eating and self-esteem predict body image dissatisfaction among obese men and women seeking bariatric surgery. *International Journal of Eating Disorders, 37*(4), 347–351.

Grilo, C. M., Masheb, R. M., Brody, M., Toth, C., Burke-Martindale, C. H., & Rothschild, B. S. (2005). Childhood maltreatment in extremely obese male and female bariatric surgery candidates. *Obesity Research, 13,* 123–130.

Harter, S., Bresnick, S., Bouchey, H. A., & Whitesell, N. R. (1997). The development of mutiple role-related selves during adolescence. *Development and Psychopathology, 9,* 835–853.

Hepertz, S., Keilmann, R., Wolf, A. M., Hedebrand, J., & Senf, W. (2004). Do psychosocial variables predict weight loss or mental health after obesity surgery? A systematic review. *Obesity Research, 12,* 1554–1569.

Holzwarth, R., Huber, D., Majkrzak, A., & Tareen, B. (April, 2002). Outcome of gastric bypass patients. *Obesity Surgery, 12*(2), 261–264.

Hsu, L. K. G., Betancourt, S., & Sullivan, S. P. (January, 1996). Eating disturbances before and after vertical banded gastroplasty: A pilot study. *International Journal of Eating Disorders, 19*(1), 23–34.

Hsu, L. K. G., Mulliken, B., McDonagh, B., Krupa Das, S., Rand, W., Fairburn, C. G., et al. (2002). Binge eating disorder in extreme obesity. *Journal of Obesity, 26*(10), 1398–1403.

Hsu, L. K. G., Sullivan, S. P., & Benotti, P. N. (1998). Eating disturbances and outcome of gastric bypass surgery: A pilot study. *International Journal of Eating Disorders, 21*(4), 385–390.

Huddleston, P. (1996). *Prepare for surgery, heal faster: A guide of mind–body techniques.* Cambridge: Angel River.

Livingston, E. H., Huerta, S., Arthur, D., Lee, S., De Shields, S., & Heber, D. (November, 2002). Male gender is a predictor of morbidity and age a predictor of mortality for patients undergoing gastric bypass surgery. *Annals of Surgery, 236*(5), 576–582.

Livingston, E. H., & Ko, C.Y. (June 1, 2002). Assessing the relative contribution of individual risk factors on surgical outcome for gastric bypass surgery: A baseline probability analysis. *Journal of Surgery Research, 105* (1), 48–52.

Maggard, M. A., Shugarman, L. R., Suttorp, M., Maglione, M., Sugerman, H. J., Livingston, E. H., et al. (2005). Meta-analysis: Surgical treatment of obesity. *Annals of Internal Medicine, 142,* 547–559.

McCullough, James P., Jr. (2000). *Treatment for chronic depression: Cognitive behavioral analysis system of psychotherapy.* New York: Guilford.

National Institutes of Health, & National Heart, Lung, and Blood Institute. (1998). *Clinical guidelines on the identification, evaluation, and treatment of overweight and obesity in adults: The evidence report.* Bethesda, MD: National Institutes of Health.

Pope, G. D., Birkmeyer, J. D., & Finlayson, S. R. (November–December, 2002). National trends in utilization and in-hospital outcomes of bariatric surgery. *Journal of Gastrointestinal Surgery, 6*(6), 855–861.

Powers, P. S., Perez, A., Boyd, F., & Rosemurgy, A. (1999). Eating pathology before and after bariatric surgery: A prospective review. *International Journal of Eating Disorders, 25,* 293–300.

Sarwer, D. B., Wadden, T. A., & Fabricatore, A. N. (2005). Psychosocial and behavioral aspects of bariatric surgery. *Obesity Research, 13,* 639–648.

Shuster, M. H., & Vazquez, J. A. (2005). Nutritional concerns related to roux-en-Y gastric bypass: What every clinician needs to know. *Critical Care Nursing Quarterly 28*(3), 227–260; quiz, 261–262.

Smith, D. E., Marcus, M. D., & Kaye, W. (1992). Cognitive-behavioral treatment of obese binge eaters. *International Journal of Eating Disorders, 12,* 257–262.

Striegel-Moore, R. H. (1993). Etiology of binge eating: A developmental perspective. In C. G. Fairburn & G. T. Wilson (Eds.), *Binge eating: Nature, assessment, and treatment* (pp. 144–172). New York: Guilford.

Tsai, A. G., & Wadden, T. A. (2005). Systematic review: an evaluation of major commercial weight loss programs in the United States. *Annals of Internal Medicine, 142*(1), 56–66.

Wadden, T. A., Sarwer, D. B., Womble, L. G., Foster, G. D., McGuckin, B. G., & Schimmel, A. (2002). Psychosocial aspects of obesity and obesity surgery. *Surgical Clinics of North America, 81*(5), 1001–1024.

Woodward, B. G. (2001). *A complete guide to obesity surgery: Everything you need to know about weight loss surgery and how to succeed.* New Bern: Trafford.

Yanovski, S. Z. (1993). Binge eating disorder: Current knowledge and future directions. *Obesity Research, 1,* 306–324.